COVID-19

LESSONS LEARNED
AND UNLEARNED

DR PATRICK CHU

*This book is dedicated to and written for all the people
who perished in this pandemic and their families*

Contents

Introduction

It was in May 2020 I had the idea of working on this book. By now, it would not be necessary for me to explain in detail what Covid-19 is. Simply put, this name was defined by the World Health Organization (WHO) as a coronavirus infection causing a severe form of viral pneumonia initially reported in the city of Wuhan in China in December 2019, thus defining and denoting an infectious disease outbreak caused by severe acute respiratory syndrome coronavirus 2 (SARS-CoV-2), which later in February 2020 was officially named as Covid-19 by the WHO. Every living person in every corner of the world now knows about Covid-19. It strikes not only fear, but also causes worldwide intense debates and uncertainties in how to deal with it. The debates have been heated and often unpleasant as politics, both national and international, invariably get entangled up in these debates. Unlike an imagined scenario of a giant asteroid from outer space hitting planet Earth, which we humans have never experienced before in an expanding universe that boasts so many galaxies, with so many stars, so many black holes and therefore so many unknowns, this Covid-19 is completely different. Whereas in the universe, we talk about massive objects bigger than planet Earth in the macroscopic world of the galaxies, Covid-19 refers to the damage done by a tiny piece of RNA in the microscopic world of the molecules. First and foremost, this damage is real and present. We are all going through the same experience, and the infection affects people of any nationality and ethnicity. Secondly, this happened at a time when we pride ourselves as masters of the universe, on our great technological, scientific, and biomedical achievements. We have even been told that before long, we can book our trip to the moon for leisure and adventures. We may move towards having a personal targeted therapy so that the cancer cells in our body can be eradicated. Our brain neurons can be kept forever young by replacing the ageing and forgetful cells with regenerative cells. These are but a few of the promising, exciting developments on the horizon. This future paints a picture for us which is beyond our imagination, and we are on the verge of seeing that imagination being turned into reality. There is a great acceleration in the practical application of our knowledge. The advances are so fast that for someone like me, in his sixties, I can justifiably feel that I may fail to catch up with society, let alone enjoy the wonderful things that society promises to bring to our lives. Meanwhile, I can also be reassured by these promises that we may have longer and longer life, for those of us who are comfortably well-off and therefore lucky enough to fund what is required. We are, or were, all caught up in the wonderful world of opportunities. I sometimes even imagine that if time could be pushed back so that I could become a kid again, a sort of real life Benjamin Button, who could start school again, then how wonderful and exciting the things I would be taught, compared with the things I was taught.

We were told that the basic rule in getting on in life is: work hard, and you shall be rewarded, assuming of course that all other factors are equal or at least comparable with each other. But of course, all factors are never equal, and that is why there are the rich, super rich, and even mega rich with wealth beyond imagination (few good people in this group are real philanthropists), the poor and the very poor, with the middle class trapped in the middle. Ironically this is just about the most suitable name assigned, accidentally, to this group of people, the middle class. The difference in income among these various groups, or income inequality, is now calibrated as the Gini index by the economists. The rich countries, according to their wealth as measured by their Gross Domestic Product (GDP), are collectively called G20 (the group of 19 wealthiest and industrialized countries in the world, plus the European Union), G8, G7 and G2. Interestingly, none of the Nordic countries are members of the G20. These rich G groups wield the most influence in world affairs and call all the shots. This grouping, which started years ago as the G7, is a sure sign that the world is getting richer, never mind the Gini index of individual countries! The theory of trickle-down economics will take care of the poorer countries – money and wealth will eventually spill over to them. To be part of this G group is what countries strive hard, and work hard, to achieve. To be in the single figure group of G is regarded as a sure sign that the country has made it to the top table in the only exclusive club that matters in the world. Strangely, I have never heard it said that there is a G1, though everyone knows which country holds G1 position. As far as I am concerned, G1 is meaningless on its own and number 1 is only meaningful when there are other numbers to go along with it, or follow behind it. Everything is relative here. Nothing is absolute. It is the ranking that matters, not the absolute position of any individual country, apart from being G1, perhaps on a perpetual basis.

That was then, the world as we knew it, before Covid-19 struck. The world since then has been turned upside down. We can be forgiven for regarding the world before Covid-19 as BC and the world after as AC. A small piece of RNA managed to come out of the blue to wreak havoc on the global stage at a speed and a scale that even this speedy, accelerating modern world could never have imagined, let alone predicted and prepared for. It was like the amalgamation of a mega tsunami, combined with a perfect storm, all formed on multiple fronts, one after another, in a matter of months, with no pause in between.

It is with the intention of taking stock of Covid-19 that this book is written. In coping with this pandemic, the world went into a near complete lockdown, fearful of both its immediate and long-term future. Opinions on every aspect of our lives were expressed. These opinions all formed part of the great debates on what should be done, what could be done, and more importantly, why some things were not done! The debates would provide us with some foresight, based on hindsight, on how to prepare ourselves for the future. These debates were extremely wide in their scopes and scales. They can happen between the public and a sovereign government, between countries, between regional blocs (the USA and Europe), and much more worrying of late, between the East and the West, by which I mean mainly between the USA and China, the G2 of this world as it currently is. The depth and the width of the debates are one which I would call a once-in-a-lifetime debate. I personally cannot recall the last occasion when there were such intensive global debates affecting nearly every aspect of our lives. Global situations as devastating as

WW1 and WW2 were not comparable in its timescale. Even the dropping of the two atomic bombs, which was perhaps more devastating but very localized, cannot be compared with Covid-19 as the destruction caused by the atomic bomb was calculated fairly accurately before its use by the atomic physicists working on it (the Manhattan Project). The decision to use it was made by men too. The carnage was national, targeted at one country. One part of the world lost while the other part of the world won.

Useful debates can often lead to balanced and measured action. It is therefore with this in mind that I feel it is appropriate that I formulate this book on these debates, with a view that out of these debates, we can all be better prepared for the next waves in the future, as surely they will come. It is just a question of when they will happen and where they will happen, in a world that is big enough to have different cultures and yet small enough for the virus to infect everyone with different cultures.

In this age of almost uncontrolled and unregulated proliferation of news and social media, news reporting and opinion-shaping often have a tendency to go for headline-grabbing sensationalism to attract readers, at the expense of objectivity and rationality. Hence for this book, I have tried to make a personal and determined effort to be as impartial and honest as possible in narrating my views, even at the expense of making the book less interesting. The idea is not to influence how others think but rather tell it as it is, and let the readers be the judge and the jury. I think it is worth my effort as Covid-19 is simply too important an event to write about otherwise.

I hope this book can play a small part in contributing to the wider ongoing global debates by explaining to the readers the nature of these debates. The information in this book is mainly based on scientific peer reviewed journals, international organizations such as the WHO, opinion leaders in institutions, published op-ed articles and reports from the international press of high repute and credibility. There will of course be differences in opinions or disagreements from the reader, which I will respect and accept, and even mistakes, for which I accept sole responsibility.

I would also draw to the attention of the readers that one of the difficulties, minor as it may seem, is for me to decide, in writing this book, when to use the past tense or the present tense, because things are moving so fast. This is just like the situation in the medical world that while it is proper for us to refer to the latest edition of a textbook, we often find that by the time the latest edition is available, some information may already be out of date due to new information emerging on a daily basis through electronic journals or professional meetings. Writing about Covid-19 fell into the same trap. Would the contents be out of date by the time this book reaches the readers? I hope it would not, and besides, the contents of the debates may still be relevant.

Finally, there is another personal reason why I pluck up enough courage and audacity to write this book. I have always thought I am a modern man, who enjoys all the things that a modern society can offer. There is a small sense of fulfilment in my professional life and there is also a blessing that I have been able to travel to many places. I have good family and friends who provide me with wonderful company. I have tried not to be complacent, not taking for granted what life has offered me. But Covid-19 is a huge emotional event for me. I experienced feelings which I never thought I would have. I had been so narrowminded to think that as a doctor, my main contribution to my profession is to help my patients, which I hope I can still do. Covid-19 transformed me. It took me out of my own bubble to look at the world. I needed to think more, a lot more than before. It has also taught me to think more for the others too, what sort of emotional state that they may have gone through. I need to try to identify with them and yet somehow I know I never could. I tell myself that I need to modify my outlook in life and start looking for the things that really matter. I need to recalibrate my life again. Kindness, generosity and tolerance mean much, much more to me than before. Such transformation is one of the reasons that has motivated me to write this book, and hopefully in doing so, a few others may make this emotional shift as well. Covid-19 changed the world. It changed me too. I am therefore very keen to share with readers these aspirations of mine. The only way I know how is to write things down, trying my best if I could, along the way. The other main reason to write this book was, since I spent six weeks working in a hospital in China to fight the outbreak and then came back to the UK to witness and then personally go through the same but more devastating crisis in the UK, I noticed the remarkable similarities in people from both countries. There was a quiet decency and serenity that I can feel. The spontaneous expression of a smile and a nod of recognition to people we don't know. Yet somehow I feel I know them, and they know me. This was a subtle display of fortitude and togetherness I never felt before. They called this the rallying round the flag effect though I see this more as a rallying round humanity effect. Crisis tends to bring the best out of people. It is for these reasons that, despite all the hurdles and challenges I mentioned in this book, I still strike an optimistic note that in the end the world can learn and unlearn from Covid-19.

CHAPTER 1

The Outbreak
– How Unique is Covid-19?

Two simple facts tell the story: the speed and the extent of the pandemic. In just nine months, from January to September 2020, the number of global infected cases has breached 30 million with a death toll of over 1 million. The epicentre started in China, then Asia, then the Middle East, then Europe, followed by the USA, South America, Central America, then Africa, India and Australia. This is a full circle. No region in the world with a thriving population is spared. These numbers keep rising and there is no end in sight to these statistics. The consensus among experts was that peaks of the outbreaks had passed in Asia from April 2020 and passed in Europe from late May 2020. Both regions have started in earnest the process of opening up from an initial lockdown position. Yet this was more like the end of the beginning and not the beginning of the end. Even in early July, the USA was still badly affected with cases of infections rising, although it hoped that the situation may begin easing off in late July. However, no one could say where or when the next wave will come, but all predict the next wave *will* come. So, in short, the day before Covid-19 and the day after will be completely different. We may have to exit from a world of great acceleration and re-enter a world of managed deceleration, a world of slowing down and great caution in protecting us from future outbreaks. How would it be different exactly we may not know for sure now, but there's no question it will be different. Going back to the systems in the old days is no longer an option. Changes, some very significant changes, would have to be made and adapted to. We need to think of how to rehabilitate our own societies to bear a remote resemblance to the way they were, and the intelligence to know that we must not forget what we have learned this time so that we will be able to deal with the next wave.

Over the past seven months, I had the chance of watching the ways events unfold globally and nationally, at a speed which I could barely keep up. I had to run just to keep up with the news. During this very same period, I spent about half the time in the UK and half in China in which six weeks were working and living in

a hospital in the city of Shenzhen, near the border with
Hong Kong. I worked seven days a week, at the height of
the crisis in China. I am a senior consultant in Hong Kong
University Shenzhen Hospital (HKU SZH). Though I can
hardly consider myself to be truly one of the courageous
frontline staff, I was nevertheless clinically responsible
for overseeing the isolation wards where all the suspected
Covid-19 patients were being managed and monitored. Such
patients were tested regularly for Covid-19, and if anyone
was tested positive then he or she would be immediately
transferred to the local infectious disease hospital for
treatment. Sometimes I had to deal with pretty tricky
situations as well. Then I came back to the UK right before
the lockdown in the UK, when it entered into the peak
of the crisis too. So my whole world, during these seven
months, was all about Covid-19, both in my professional life
and in my personal life.

There will be many, of course, and indeed very
necessary and timely, scientific papers, scholarly work
and books, of great merits and value, coming out soon, in
different languages in different parts of the world. These
are hugely anticipated and must also be welcome. There
should be no prejudice involved. Every individual or
country can have a legitimate right to have a say. This is a
global crisis. The stakes are simply much too high to allow
any room for prejudice as this is a war against a piece of

RNA which does not differentiate between nationalities, ethnicities or social classes. It goes where it wants to go, as long as we allow it to go. The world must come up with a checkmate where no further move is possible. Either we win or the whole world loses. The process towards achieving the right result for us can of course be long or short, depending on how smart, and how collaborative we are, on a global basis. This process does not depend on, thankfully, how smart the opponent is, as it only moves one way. Therefore, the more knowledge we have and agreed actions there are, the better placed the world will be in dealing with the next wave.

During these months, I have seen a lot, experienced a lot and above all read a lot. Much of the information I read is valuable, and there are new lessons to be learned while some old orthodoxy needs to be unlearned. Regrettably also, some of what I have read was hearsay or half informed opinions. In these days of crisis, opinions can vary widely. At best, it is like a good detective fiction or first-rate investigative journalism, with the good intentions of bringing and piecing every bit of information together, chronologically, meaningfully and rationally. This can then be used as the basis of forming a good and well considered policy. Setting up an effective policy can only be done if various key facts are known, unknowns are known, data are clarified, public needs are identified and implementable in a way which is beneficial and affordable to all. Speed and nuances are required but equally hastiness must be avoided. Another key function of these views and opinions is that it can form a very useful basis for an all-rounded public debate. However, there were opinions which were cynical in nature, disguised and expressed as tools for the purpose of willful disinformation, with ill-conceived intention. This is mischief of the worst form. Such misinformation or disinformation is sadly becoming a noticeable development in politics of the world today, known as the modern post-truth world, with the disappearance of shared objective standards for 'truth' and the 'circuitous slippage between facts or alternate facts, knowledge, opinion, belief, and truth'.

The mischief, such as it is, can often be part of a well-coordinated, politically motivated misinformation campaign with the sole purpose of claiming credit or blaming others. We are all, without exception, currently fighting against an invisible piece of RNA, and we must never allow it to be turned into a battle in which we are fighting against each other. To me, there will be no greater sin if this is allowed to happen and become part of an agenda to cloud our judgment on how best to help our fellow human beings. Countries and institutions in the world must come together; a global crisis needs a global solution.

CHAPTER 2

The Clinical Spectrum of the Infection

Covid-19, as defined by the WHO, is caused by a specific virus belonging to the group called Coronavirus family of viruses that cause diseases mainly in mammals and birds, especially bats. This Covid-19 virus has made the jump from animals to humans, in a biological process called zoonosis.

The word 'corona' is derived from the Greek word meaning 'crown'. This is because, under electron microscopy, the infective part of the virus, known as virions, appears as a fringe of bulbous surface projections creating an image similar to a crown. In Ancient Greece when someone was crowned, the crown would have flower-like petals looking like bulbous projections.

Just like the rhinovirus group of viruses (rhino means nose in Greek) or the influenza virus, this Covid-19 virus attacks our respiratory system from the nose, the throat, trachea and bronchus all the way down to the smallest of lung cells called alveoli, where through these cells oxygen from the air enters into our blood and where carbon dioxide exits from our blood, then through the airway back into the air. So, in order for the alveoli to do their work, which is called gaseous exchange, we need to breathe in and breathe out to ensure a constant supply of oxygen. The rhinovirus and influenza virus affect mainly the nose, throat and even the trachea. This disease is usually commonly known by the public and the medical fraternity as a slightly different term called the upper respiratory tract infection (URTI). This is also sometimes known as a 'cold like' illness, or the common cold, with mild symptoms like sneezing, nasal congestion or a runny nose. The vast majority of those affected recover within days, without any significant short or long-term complications. The flu virus generally causes more systemic symptoms than the rhinovirus, with additional symptoms such as fever, cough, muscle and joint pain, and it may travel down further along the respiratory tract to reach the alveoli, causing pneumonia. All these flu-like systemic symptoms such as joint pain, muscle pain or fever are not caused by direct damage to the body by the viruses but the body's immune and inflammatory response to fight off the virus. In other words, these systemic symptoms are side effects of our body's fight against these viruses, which is why taking tablets like aspirin can help to relieve the symptoms even though aspirin does not have a direct effect on the virus. These symptoms suggest our bodies are producing antibodies to fight off the flu virus, and the symptoms are resolved when the battle is won.

However, more severe forms of illness can be caused by this group of coronaviruses as they move down the respiratory track to the alveoli, where the process of oxygenation at the cellular level is disrupted or destroyed. This is what Covid-19 virus can do to us. Both the SARS (Severe Acute Respiratory Syndrome) epidemic in Southern China, especially Hong Kong in 2003, and the MERS (Middle East Respiratory Syndrome) outbreak in 2012 were severe infections as these viruses spread along the whole respiratory tract causing coughs along the way (as the body tried to cough to expel the viruses in droplets – that is why it can be so contagious), and made their way to the alveoli where they can do most damage, leading to failure of oxygenation, called respiratory failure in common terms. This is the most severe form of damage and can even be life threatening. It is the main reason why these three viruses are so feared because all of them, in attacking the lungs, can lead to respiratory failure and become life threatening without ventilator support. The severely affected patients will be gasping for breath, as the struggling and damaged alveoli can no longer get the oxygen.

Covid-19 is different to these two other coronaviruses in that the spectrum of the disease is broad, with around 80% of cases having mild infection (some of these may be asymptomatic), 15% being severe infection requiring oxygen therapy, and the remaining 5% being more critical cases needing ICU (Intensive Care Unit) level of care. This is why it can initially, at the outset of symptoms, be confused with the seasonal flu. There may also be many people carrying the disease and displaying no symptoms, making it even harder to control. These asymptomatic cases were estimated to range from as high as 25% to 40%, of those tested positive for this virus. This is truly alarming as it actually means that there may be 25% of those affected by this virus who will not know they are carrying this virus, and without being tested, normal life continues for them. This will be the rich seeds in spreading the disease to others.

Most worryingly, the concoction of symptoms of fever, dry cough, shortness of breath and abnormal changes of Chest CT can equally and indeed more commonly be due to other pathogens such as bacteria. This is why it is so important to establish the proper diagnosis of Covid-19 as the actual cause of the virus pneumonia, to be differentiated from bacteria pneumonia which is far less transmissible while at the same time more treatable by antibiotics. This differentiation is usually possible by sending a throat swab from the patient to the laboratory for the detection of the presence of Covid-19 through the presence of its RNA or sending the sputum samples of a patient for the presence of bacteria through the presence of its growth in culture.

Much is still not known about the clinical variants of this virus infection. It has been suggested that there may be other target organs for damage such as the heart, the kidney, the gastrointestinal tract, the liver or even the central nervous system. The list grows longer with time, such as loss of sense of taste or smell, or the development of a severe inflammation of the blood vessels called Kawasaki's Disease, especially in children. The data on these are still being collected.

Around 15% to 20% of Covid-19 cases are classed as 'severe'. Severity means patients who have breathing difficulty, with low oxygen level in their blood, needing hospitalization and oxygen therapy. Some of these affected patients may even require intensive care (ICU) if ventilatory support is needed. These most severe cases, needing ICU, accounts for about 5% of cases. The current death rate of the severe infection varies between 0.7% and 3.4% depending on whether the patients have any co-morbid conditions and more importantly, the access to ventilator support and crucially, access to intensive care units. As more information is now available there are now early indications that the clinical spectrum can be much wider and unpredictable. It is not possible, at this stage, for doctors to have a grasp on the extent of the damage that Covid-19 can cause in any affected individual. We even do not know with any degree of certainty if it can recur in a patient who is thought to have recovered. In other words, can a recovered patient develop a relapse in the absence of re-infection?

Furthermore, there is no specific treatment currently available. As a result, the current worldwide clinical effort in this respect is mainly through clinical trials to see if any other existing antiviral treatment drugs can be effective in treating Covid-19. There have also been talks floating around about the use of hydroxychloroquine, which is mainly used to treat certain types of malaria or arthritis. This drug appeared to offer some hope in some cases, but so far it has not been proven to be significantly clinically useful to be recommended for general use. Yet, the fearful state of the public was such that in April, when the information of its possible use was first mentioned in the public media, the world supply of this drug immediately went under severe strain due to the intense public demand for it. This has a knock-on effect for those non-Covid-19 patients who really need the drug, which is basically used to treat some form of malaria and severe arthritis of an autoimmune nature (this means the body produces antibodies on its own accord, which may in turn cause damage to the joints, the skin, the blood and the kidneys). By late May 2020, it had been shown in clinical trials in both the USA and the UK that it was not effective. The other drug which seemed to have shown clinical efficacy, especially in the early infective phase, is remdesivir. This is an antiviral drug which was first used to treat patients with Ebola virus infection in West Africa with some benefits. However, this drug was not developed extensively by the pharmacological industry following the resolution of the Ebola outbreak in West Africa. It remained very much on the shelf, but not in the production line. Still, because it is an antiviral drug, it remains the frontrunner in the race for a specific antiviral treatment. There were recent clinical studies which showed that this drug, used in the early stage of the disease, can possibly shorten the duration of infection. Many clinical trials for this drug are still ongoing, and we will not need to wait for too long, possibly six months, before further proof of its clinical validity may come through. There are other major clinical trials, using a combination (a cocktail of antiviral drugs) of therapy, based on much like the approach used successfully in the treatment for HIV infection currently. The principle here is to eradicate the virus by attacking it on multiple levels. In addition, there were also clinical results coming out in July 2020 showing that interferon-beta can also be used as a possible effective treatment for Covid-19. It is anticipated that validated clinical results of these various forms of treatment, or combination of treatments, will start to emerge in late 2020 or early 2021. Another main area of active research is the development of a vaccine to prevent the disease. In the race on research for new treatments for Covid-19 by drugs or prevention of Covid-19 by vaccines, the four most important factors to consider by the scientists, doctors, manufacturers and the marketing experts are efficacy, safety, production capacity, and cost/affordability to meet the global demand, both for the current crisis and for the future waves.

Since currently there is no proven antiviral treatment to treat individual patients infected with Covid-19 or vaccine available to protect the public from developing the disease, the only treatment approach that we can adopt will be supportive in nature such as the use of artificial ventilators if and when the lung damage is significant. Even this approach is faced with huge challenges. For a start, the ventilators must be available when and where they are needed. Secondly, there is no consensus about when to use ventilators or when to transfer the patients to the ICU (intensive care unit). The decision is often left to the senior clinicians in respiratory medication. Therefore, it is dependent on the clinical opinions of the experts in a particular hospital. While this may provide uniformity within a hospital, there is still much debate on the formulation of acceptable and agreed national or even international guidelines for all to follow, particularly on the admission criteria to the ICU. The intense global debate currently undertaken can possibly lead to a better clinical algorithm which most, if not all, can follow. This clinical benchmark and standard are very important as it has been estimated that the severe cases (those which require ventilatory support) may be as high as 20% of the infected cases and the mortality rate of those in the ICU can be as high as 30%. The overall mortality of all the infected cases is around 3.4%, based on the WHO estimates released in early April. This is high compared with a mortality of less than 1% caused by seasonal flu. So, the epidemiology and the clinical spectrum of Covid-19 are different from seasonal flu, contrary to what some people seemed to have suggested in the early phase of the outbreak.

Given the huge and unprecedented effort put in globally to fight this virus, led by countries such as the USA, China, the European Union and the UK, I am reasonably hopeful that within the next 12-18 months, a cocktail of specific antiviral treatment or prevention by a vaccine, both of proven value, will be available. But until then, we must still keep our vigilance, as we currently are, in protecting ourselves. This self-protection is actually one of the most important aspects of protection from the virus. The efficacy and importance of hand washing and matters of personal hygiene cannot be overemphasized. Simple and proper hand washing with soap is often very effective to kill off the virus from our hands. As the portal of entry is mainly through inhalation of droplets either via the nose or the mouth, wearing masks is also an effective means, which some in the West still need to be convinced of. The droplets can also enter via the mucous membrane of the eyes, so wearing goggles or installation of a plastic barrier as a mechanical shield can help too. These, what I called the triads of personal measures – frequent handwashing, wearing masks, and wearing goggles – are easy to implement and relatively cheap. The cost benefits ratio is overwhelmingly weighted in favour of these measures. No wonder that there was a shortage of masks initially in China and other Asian countries and later the acute shortage of masks in the West, as everyone was chasing these to protect themselves.

One debate which is stimulating much interest is the gender difference in mortality. This observation seems to have been confirmed in many countries with elderly male patients with co-morbid conditions being particularly vulnerable. This cannot be explained currently but one

postulation which may be gaining ground is that females
have an extra X chromosome with a chromosomal
makeup of XX while males have one X chromosome
less with a chromosomal makeup of XY. This difference
may have a biological significance according to the
Darwinian theory of evolution and survival advantage.
An extra X chromosome in the female will ensure that any
newborn will either have an XX or XY chromosome as its
chromosomal makeup, thus guaranteeing that the child
will inherit half of the genetic material from the biological
father and half of the genetic material from the biological
mother. The lack of an extra X chromosome in male
biologically probably makes the male stronger physically
as the male produces more testosterone. On the other
hand, the extra X chromosome may enhance the capacity
of immunity in the females. A number of critical immune
genes are located in the X chromosome and in particular a
gene which codes for a protein called TLR7, which detects
single stranded RNA like the coronavirus. As a result
of the extra X chromosome, this protein is expressed at
twice the dose on the immune cells in the females. In
other words, there is possible immune amplification in the
female. In addition, we know that our natural immunity
declines with age, so it may be that this presence of only
one X chromosome in the male may reduce the immunity
capacity in the male, compared with the female, especially

when the male starts to age. In other words, there is a theory that males may be immunologically less robust and responsive than females, thus making man more susceptible to an attack from a virus from which the body depends almost exclusively on the immunity response to produce the necessary antibodies in sufficient quantities to fight off the virus.

Another worrying and surprising observation which is generating much debate is the significant difference in mortality between countries. The USA, the richest country in the world, has the highest number of affected cases and death toll from Covid-19 infection. This is followed by Western European countries such as the UK, Spain and Italy. These countries also have a high number of deaths. And yet countries in Asia such as China, Japan and South Korea all have much lower numbers of deaths, adjusted for population and infection rate. This debate has ascended to a higher political level as it was regarded as a marker for national success and pride, which of course should not be the case. Whether the difference is true or not, only time and further analysis can tell. Crude comparison at this stage of an incomplete story is not scientific, especially since each country may record and analyse its deaths differently. Many epidemiologists attribute this difference to the practice of extensive testing, contact tracing, severe restrictions and lockdown approach. The lockdown approach, in particular, was a globally unprecedented measure first undertaken by China in the city of Wuhan and then the province of Hubei, where the first outbreak occurred. The lower death toll can also mean the Asian countries may be much better prepared in dealing with Covid-19, having themselves gone through the trauma of SARS in 2003 and MERS in 2015. Take Hong Kong, for example: by the middle of June 2020 the death toll in Hong Kong from Covid-19 was only five, in a city with a population of about 7.5 million! This was a figure that any city or country would die for. One of the main reasons is that the level of personal hygiene and the awareness of the importance of public health in a densely urban population has been raised to a much higher level since SARS. Basic public health measures such as clean toilets, clean markets, handwashing, and wearing of masks in any epidemic have become a matter of course and good habits. These good practices are practised throughout the city from the hospitals, to schools, to clinics, to health centres, and most importantly, to the care homes too, where the rapidly ageing population turns to for help. My own view is, personal as it is, that better preparedness can help mainly in the reduction of number of infective cases but not necessarily lead to a lower death toll. Death from Covid-19 depends on many other factors, not least the equitable access to medical care, the use of tests, and protective gear for staff. I also suspect that the difference in mortality may be explainable possibly by a different and far more complex interplay of genetic, ethnicity and environmental factors, which can be significantly different among the indigenous people from the USA, Europe and Asian countries. For example, a neurological condition called multiple sclerosis, is a fairly common neurological condition in the West and yet very rare in the East. Another condition called the inflammatory bowel disease (IBS) is common in the West and previously rare in the East, but with globalization and the change in lifestyle and diets, this IBS is now being more and more recognized in China. And in our own hospital, HKU SZH, we even have a specialist clinic for it.

By late April 2020, people started to debate how we should interpret the death toll in order to truly understand the clinical severity of the Covid-19 infection. Up till then, the daily reports in the UK were mainly on Covid-19 related deaths in hospitals. This kind of reporting was used by many other countries too. We did not know if elderly people living in care homes have a similar mortality compared with their counterparts either in hospitals or their own homes. The intuition here was that the more severe cases must be in the hospitals. This possible difference in institutional mortalities posed a real question which cannot be explained by the simple assumption that the elderly have more co-morbid conditions. The difference in death rates in this respect needs a better scientific explanation and answer. We need to know if those who reside or work in the care homes are particularly vulnerable and if so, what was the extent of the problem and why? Most advanced economies all share the same demographic time bomb of an ageing population. The sooner we come up with the answer, the better our future will be served. One important way to establish this is that in order to unearth the true meaning of the number of deaths published on a daily basis, one has to look at the long term trend, then compare that with historical data. A daily death number was easy to read and made good headlines, but it was also a rather crude measure to assess the real significance of Covid-19 in any given country, let alone among countries. There are currently no international studies on how death was being recorded in different countries. We need to ascertain if the data are comparable before we come up with a more assured conclusion. Headlines are there to inform and alert us. Only comparable data can lead us to reach the right conclusion. Furthermore, it is entirely consistent with the nature of a pandemic that the location of the epicentre changed with time. In this global crisis, it was obviously clear that different countries were hit with their peaks at different times. For instance, the peak was reached in Italy just when the peak was subsiding in China. The peak was reached in the UK when Italy passed its peak.

Given this variation, the real significance of the Covid-19 related death toll in each country can only be worked out over a much longer timeframe, using the adjusted death rate methodology. This is done by looking at the standardized death rate for each country over a number of years before and after Covid-19 so that the excess death rate associated with the virus in a particular period, for instance, April 2020, can be worked out. This is commonly known as the excess death rate. Only epidemiologists and statisticians have the expertise and data to work that out. This is why modern countries have an office for national statistics which can be charged with this task. The use of big data can also help, but it will take time to get the proper information. In short, while we learn to cope with the clear and present danger of Covid-19, the real mortality rate can only be ascertained on a longer timeframe.

By the middle of May 2020, England's Office for National Statistics (ONS) has revealed that the excess deaths (deaths over and above the normal) in England and Wales in the Covid-19 pandemic topped 50,000, a much higher figure than the government's own figure, which at the time stood at 32,065! The ONS quoted that in the week ending on May 1, there had been 17,953 deaths in England and Wales (the ONS does not cover data from Scotland and Northern Ireland), 8,012 higher than the average of the past five years for that week. By July, 2020, the ONS updated

the figures to show that the excess death in England and
Wales from January to June 2020 was the highest in Europe
with an increased death rate, compared with previous
years, of 7.5%. The main reason for this was deaths in the
care homes. It was found that deaths related to Covid-19
were three times that of non-Covid-19 related deaths in
care homes. This was a shocking finding, devastating to all
and caused a national uproar. No sane society can tolerate
such a difference in health outcome. The elderly people
in care homes, albeit with co-morbid conditions, suffered,
through no fault of their own, a higher chance of death if
they have the Covid-19 infection. This also means, from
an epidemiological point of view, that those who reside
in care homes and more disturbingly, those who care for
them (the care workers), dispersed all over the society, may
be a seed for future infections, unless urgent measures
such as testing are employed to help and identify them.
This excess death toll in the care homes in the UK at the
time represented possibly the highest in Europe. Later, the
same observation of excess death toll in care homes was
also found in the USA and some other European countries
such as Belgium, Sweden, and France. For the UK, the
implication for this was huge. Right from the beginning of
dealing with the peaking of the crisis, the UK government
was so concerned in avoiding the hospital medical services
being overwhelmed that hospital beds were freed up by

discharging elderly too early to care homes without proper prior preparation, and also the care homes might have been pressured into not sending their residents to the hospital when hospital care was needed. For some elderly, hospital care, even though it may not stop the inevitability of death, can help by providing better and expert-led care in terms of symptoms relief and palliation. There were even stories of ambulance staff refusing to take calls from care homes or designated general practitioners (GPs) not visiting patients at care homes at all, relying instead solely on telemedicine. Furthermore, it was also revealed that there was a woeful lack of tests and PPEs, let alone clinical supervision, so those who were residents and workers in the care homes were completely exposed. In one private 40-bedded nursing home in a remote village in the West of Scotland, only seven of its 40 patients were spared the Covid-19 infection and at least a quarter of them had Covid-19 related death. Can this observation be seen as deliberately shifting the death from the hospital setting to the care home setting, so that beds and capacity of the NHS hospital services were protected at the expense of the care homes? The worried public was starting to wonder if the care homes were sacrificed to avoid overloading the NHS. Part of the pointer to this suggestion was that the hospital non-Covid-19 death rate during this period was lower by comparison. This was a national scandal on which there were heated parliamentary debates. Since then, the daily report from the government has started to include deaths from care homes as well.

This care home issue first reported in the UK must be addressed with the help of experts in statistics and epidemiology through a comprehensive and detailed data analysis, to prepare the communities to deal better when the next wave arrives. The public has a right to know and demand proper action on this. In contrast, no death was reported in the care homes in Hong Kong, which has a far more acute problem with an ageing population. The success in Hong Kong was due to the experience it obtained during the SARS outbreak in 2003, after which all care homes in Hong Kong have to practise regular infection control drills in coping with an outbreak three times a year with full PPEs. For them, it is a routine and standard practice. The UK and the other Western countries may take heed of the lessons learned in Hong Kong.

To round off this chapter, mention has to be made about the announcement by the UK government on June 16, 2020 of the result of a clinical trial conducted by Oxford University called the Recovery Trial. The trial is a national trial involving 175 NHS (National Health Service) hospitals in the UK with about 11,500 patients consenting to enter into the trial, in which there were various arms of drug(s) treatments. The results, at the time of writing this manuscript, were not yet published in peer reviewed journals, but it was felt that it was of such crucial public and international importance that it was announced on national TV. This is the biggest clinical trial of its kind in the world in just the three months during which the UK was going through the crisis. That the UK was able to do this remarkable trial is simply due to the fact that the NHS is a single organization funded by the public through general taxation so all hospitals in this trial in effect belong to a single organization. In other words, one single command and control centre. The drug involved in particular is an old but useful drug called dexamethasone, which has been in existence for about 60 years. It is extremely cheap and is a generic drug, so there is no patent on this drug. There were about 2,000 patients in a treatment arm to receive this drug compared to the other arm for patients which did not receive this drug. This Recovery Trial was led by Oxford University which had to terminate this treatment arm on June 12, 2020 because they had found that for those 2,000 patients who received this drug, compared with about 4,000 patients who did not receive this drug, there was a significant difference in mortality. For those patients whose infection was severe enough to be cared for in the ICU, the risk of death in those who were given a 10-day course of dexamethasone was reduced by 35% and for those who were cared for in the wards but needed oxygen therapy, the risk of death was reduced by 20%. This was a remarkable finding as it is the first time ever it has been demonstrated in a clinical trial setting that a particular form of treatment has been shown to reduce the risk of death. It is all the more remarkable because it also means that it can be used globally as the drug is so easily and cheaply available, to both rich and poor countries. The example was so quoted by the lead investigators in the trial that if this drug was used to treat eight patients in the ICU suffering from Covid-19, there would be one life saved, and the total cost of this drug in all eight patients was about GBP 40! Furthermore, no manufacturer in the world holds a monopoly on this drug. Such is the global significance of its importance that this is the first time in my whole professional career that a government announced a clinical trial result without first publishing it in a peer reviewed journal. The WHO hailed this next day as: a lifesaving scientific breakthrough. It also indicated its intention to recommend this treatment in its next global update on treatment for Covid-19 infection. I have absolutely no doubt that other institutions in countries such as the US, China, Germany or Japan have already been embarking on treatment involving this drug since the outbreak too. It is hoped that further results will start to emerge on the efficacy of this drug from these countries. It should also be emphasized that this drug is found to be effective only in those who need oxygen therapy in the ward or cared for in the ICU. In other words, it needs not be used in patients with mild symptoms and who do not have respiratory difficulty.

How can one explain this? As a practising clinician who uses the drug quite often in the care of my patients with haematological cancers, maybe I can forward a possible explanation. When a group of cells in our body get injured and die from injury, in this case Covid-19 damages the alveoli in our lungs, the virus itself and the associated cell deaths will trigger off what is known as an inflammatory response. This response is important as it is part of the healing, or cell recovery, process. These processes are mediated by biological response modifiers called cytokines, which are produced in our own bodies. This is very much similar to the same reason why we may have joint pains or muscle pains when we have the classical flu, as it is these cytokines which cause us the pain. However, occasionally, a virus infection, for some still unknown reason, can trigger off an exaggerated inflammatory response releasing too much cytokines. In other words, it becomes a case of overkill, called a cytokines storm, and once this happens, more cellular damage and death can occur. The net result is that cell deaths and inflammations are all mixed in together to perpetuate further cellular damages in a vicious cycle. This is where dexamethasone comes in, because this is a drug whose main action is to suppress inflammation and thus can help to alleviate the cytokines storm by breaking up the vicious cycle. In my own specialty, we use dexamethasone often for this purpose. It has to be said that this drug should and can only be used under supervision of specialists as it is not without side effects, though most of the side effects are manageable as the experience of using this drug has been accumulated for about 60 years.

CHAPTER 3

The Contribution of Epidemiological Debates

In general, epidemiology refers to a branch of medicine that deals with the incidence and prevalence of diseases in a defined population. It also has a role in advising and educating the public, leading to better control of the disease, and in some cases, linking these together with other factors such as genetic or environmental, in a way that will contribute to a better health outcome. In other words, it would help to improve the overall health status of a society or country. A classic example would be the effects of smoking. It has long been confirmed from epidemiological studies that smoking was directly linked to cancer of the lungs and cardiovascular problems, which was proved consistently for decades. Yet the scientific findings and the public health implications, not to mention the addictive nature of smoking, were initially not widely known. The tobacco companies tried to suppress the information and even smeared the epidemiological findings. When finally it went to the US Supreme Court as a case of class action against the tobacco companies, the verdict was one of the biggest punitive actions against giant commercial companies in corporate history, despite these giants spending an enormous amount of money in lobbying for political favours and fighting the court case. This illustrates clearly the role of epidemiology in tackling diseases, no matter what the odds are against its success. Furthermore, in our modern age of modelling and big data, the role of epidemiology can assume more importance and the information it provides can be more scientifically valid and powerful.

This branch of medicine is particularly useful in infectious diseases where no one, however good their living habits are, is exempted. For instance, it has enabled us to be more aware of the extent of the health impact with the emerging problems of drug resistance in some cases of TB, HIV, and hepatitis. It is because of the very importance of epidemiology and surveillance of diseases that one of the first things the United Nations did was to set up the World Health Organization (WHO) in 1948.

As for Covid-19, because of its unprecedented speed

of spread, which is directly related to the transmissibility and the infectivity of the virus, the world of epidemiology has gone into overdrive. All the data have to be collected, verified, analysed and updated to enable the state of the global crisis to reflect the situation in real time. In epidemiology, one of the main tools in its skills set is modelling. Modelling is a bit like the weather forecast; it cannot be 100% accurate, but based on a combination of mathematical calculations, meteorological and historical data, it can give us an indicative predictor of when and where a storm brewing up in the oceans is heading our way. In many respects, epidemiology works very much on the same principle. Remodelling the modelling is required, with constant updating and monitoring of the latest information and data. This can provide the public and the policymakers with the timely, relevant and accurate information on the pandemic, thus enabling the politicians, the doctors, the scientists and the public to make proper policies and preparations, or adjust existing policies.

The task has become exceptionally more important, urgent and challenging in Covid-19 because of the lack of effective antiviral treatments of infection or vaccines for the prevention of infection. Previous experience in SARS, MERS and Ebola outbreaks may help but this Covid-19 was the first real pandemic, unlike the three previous outbreaks which were primarily regional in nature.

One of the first challenges was that the prevalence of the virus was not really known since the outbreak only started in December 2019. There simply was not enough data within such a short time on a global scale to work out a proper estimate of its prevalence. For example, one of the estimates showed that the rate of asymptomatic carriers, that is, people who have the infection, thus carrying the virus, without being affected by it and therefore could spread the disease without knowing that themselves, could be as high as 25%. The term super carriers is sometimes used to describe some in this group. The presence of this group, quantitatively undefinable and undetectable, unless by tests, at any particular time, can be very worrying as this will enable the infection to spread unchecked. This leaves us to deal, without any other option, only with the consequences of infection and not particularly effective in dealing with its prevention. Only a very large population-based study, with good screening blood tests to ascertain the presence of the virus or antibodies against the virus, can yield this vital piece of information. To obtain such information requires some very top-notch population profile studies involving careful planning, execution, data collection and data analysis. It cannot be achieved overnight just by pouring resources into it.

The second challenge is to know the infectivity or the transmissibility of this virus. Here the epidemiologists used the R value, which is the basic reproduction value describing the average number of people whom an individual patient carrying the virus can infect. So, by definition, the R value in a non-infective disease is naturally zero. In highly infectious diseases, the R value becomes a very important figure. It can be used also as a crude benchmark to test how effective (a downward trend towards 1 and then maintained at below 1) the infection is coming under control with various measures or how ineffective these measures are (an upward trend from 1). It is also an indicator useful for day-to-day and week-to-week information. For instance, if the R value is 3, it means that someone with this infection can spread this infection to three people. Of course, this is not an absolute guide as the infectivity can vary based on other factors, such as personal habits, close physical contact or the environment. A person who works as a lone gardener in a private, detached house with a large garden in rural England probably has a lower R value than a person selling hot dogs in more crowded areas where human traffics are higher. Nevertheless, the R value is still a good indicator, assuming all other conditions are matched or factored in, not least because it can be easily understood by the public in assessing the severity of the outbreak. For Covid-19, the WHO estimated in March 2020 that the R value was between 2 and 2.5. By comparison, the seasonal flu has an R value of 1.3 while measles has a higher

R value of 12-18.

For the UK, the R value during the peak of the crisis in the middle of April 2020 was estimated to be at 3-4.6, which was a higher figure than the WHO suggested as an average on a global basis. It indicated almost certainly that a more serious crisis was in the making and so the UK government set a target of getting the R value of being consistently under 1 as one of the key performance indicators. By mid-May, just over six weeks of social isolation and lockdown of all non-essential services, the R value came down to around 0.7-0.9. It does need to be stressed that this R value is only a measurement of its infectivity but not how deadly the infection may be.

The third key area where the science of epidemiology will be of great value is contact tracing and population surveillance. The rationale for this is self-explanatory and intuitive but the logistics of implementing this are very difficult. Even though it is important to do, various countries vary widely in their ability to implement this. The main reason for the difficulty is that the first hurdle to overcome is the ability to scale up the tests so massively to almost an equivalence of testing for a population profile. It is costly and many countries simply do not have the testing ability and capacity of such an endeavour. In this area, China is leading the effort because of its ability to carry out the test in approved laboratories and hospitals dotted around the whole country. The second hurdle is that it must be part of a government sponsored and initiated public health programme. Private purchase, over the counter, of self-testing commercial kits simply would not do. In the West, even if a country is hoping to carry out this study for the benefits of the population, it may still run into problems as some would argue that there would need to be a balance between individual privacy and public safety. The best way to carry out such a contact tracing and surveillance programme is to start it as a properly-funded, scientific-led national or international epidemiological study, preferably with the latter under the auspices of the WHO. All ethical issues and the consenting processes in any study must be fully resolved before it can be started. In my view, this is quite possibly the most important study as this is the only way to know the prevalence of the virus in a given population at any given time. This would also tell us how many people within this group may already have immunity from past infection. International study such as this, coordinated by the WHO, will also help the less well-off countries in continents such as those in Africa and the Middle East. High prevalence may tell us about the potential extent of the problem while high immunity may tell us the extent of our protection. Similar population-based studies have been done regularly before. For instance, breast screening for cancer was started more than

20 years ago, and colonoscopy screening for bowel cancer was started 10 years ago, both for the early detection of cancers and for study on their prevalence.

In most countries, the peak lasts about six to eight weeks, then it starts to wear off as a result of a multitude of measures such as isolation, social distancing, testing, contact tracing, access to medical care, wearing of masks and frequent hand washing. In the UK, the first items that were snapped up to the point of no supplies were hand sanitizers and toilet paper, not to mention that masks were never on the shelf in the first place! These measures were all part of the efforts which the epidemiologists term as 'flattening the curve'. The peak would not pass without the acceptance and active compliance of the people. In countries like China (including Hong Kong and Macau) and South Korea, the measures undertaken there were decisive, speedy and daring, as the people there still could remember the traumatic and devastating experience of the SARS epidemic in 2003. Real lessons were learned then. For Covid-19, China was the first country to experience it and also the first country to come out of it, coping admirably well up to the present time. Where there are some sporadic new cases, the local government and health bureaus took decisive and immediate measures, as in some areas of Beijing in June 2020. The precautionary measures such as massive screening by tests, surveillance, contact tracing and

isolation of suspected cases in China are now very much
in place, ready for the early detection of the arrival of the
second wave. I think on this, China is leading the rest of the
world. One very novel way of looking at it was devised and
published by Oxford University in the UK. The researchers
at Oxford University used matrix of data by the measures
undertaken by the governments to test for the effectiveness
of government lockdown in what is now known as the
world's first stringency index, using various indicators
including school closures, work closures and travel bans.
It was not a surprise that some countries in Asia scored
very high in this stringency index, while the UK scored
just above the average. India also scored very high as India
imposed a quarantine of 21 days, in contrast with the 14
days that most countries used.

Another area of interesting debates, still very unresolved,
is the difference in the practice of extensive and frequent
temperature checks in Asian countries such as China, South
Korea and Japan in the East, as opposed to most countries
in the West. This is usually done by hand-held non-contact
temperature monitors in airports, all subways, entrances
to any malls, hospitals and border checkpoints. Any visitor
from overseas will undoubtedly be familiar with it. I tend
to wear a cap when I travel these days, but I habitually and
automatically remove my cap when I pass through any
border control in China just so the monitor can point at

my forehead and check my temperature out! In the past, I was often reminded to remove the cap and now it is a well practised habit for me. The debate for its use is mainly on the point that some patients, even if infected, would not have a fever. Furthermore, the fever could be circadian in nature, and thus bears no relation to the time of entry at a certain point in time. Besides, the accuracy of these hand-held monitors, though easy to use (no training is required) may be overestimated, thus it can lead to a false sense of security. It has been pointed out often by the antagonists of the use of these hand-held monitors that the first patient outside China was a patient who travelled from Wuhan to Thailand in January 2020 where there were already temperature checks for all passengers at exit points from China and entry points in Thailand, but the patient still passed through the temperature checkpoint for the simple reason that she had no fever at the time. Yet, the routine check of temperature cannot be completely discarded; it is a clear message that everyone should be vigilant and if one has a fever, then one should not venture out. Just the other day, after the UK started to gradually open up its retail sector, I went to the local Apple shop. I had to queue up and then when it was my turn, my temperature was checked before I was allowed to go in. So whatever the merits, this is now a standard practice, and I am convinced that no one was complaining about its necessity.

CHAPTER 4

The Debate on Herd Immunity

With all the new terms coming out from this pandemic, herd immunity is by far the most controversial and deserves some explanation. The words were first used in public in the UK press when it reported that the UK government's initial response was to move towards an achievement of herd immunity, which in simple terms, means to acquire natural immunity by the masses through exposure to the virus and subsequent development of antibodies against this virus. The thinking for this Darwinian approach is that since the virus pandemic has happened and it was much too late to stop it, and since the mortality is reasonably low especially in the young, it may be an option that, if the society lets the virus run its course, as it will, then at the end of this process most people, called the herd, would have acquired the immunity to protect this herd and to prevent them from spreading infection to others.

It then follows that the attainment of such a herd immunity will be beneficial in the long term in any given population but it does mean more people will suffer, perhaps even die from the infection in the short term if this pandemic was allowed to run its course, as it takes time for herd immunity to develop. During this period, many of those exposed would have to bear the risk of being symptomatic before immunity can be developed. It is estimated that the level of herd immunity should be around 60% to 70% of the population for this to be a safe, effective and acceptable way to contain any second or future waves of infection. This school of thought advocates that since resources are stretched and limited, it is better to have a graded and calibrated response to identify, isolate and protect the vulnerable groups. Those vulnerable ones are the elderly, the very young, and those with co-morbid medical conditions. It is like a risk-stratified, age-based and targeted approach. Meanwhile, let the healthy and the young develop this herd immunity, through mild or asymptomatic infection. However, this will mean the young and healthy are allowed to take the risk of an infection, the science of which we don't really know that well. We certainly don't know the extent of its clinical diversity.

We are therefore stepping into various unknowns, and therefore morally unacceptable. The counter alternative in contrast to this herd immunity approach is the mainstream school of thought, adopted by many countries. It is known as the total lockdown approach to break the transmission, initiated in January 2020 in the city of Wuhan in China, when the Chinese government realized that there was a severe outbreak to deal with. This lockdown approach claimed success in barely just under 10 weeks. Both schools of thoughts are plausible: herd immunity may show long-term gain while the lockdown approach may be unsustainable in the long term, though the lockdown approach undoubtedly will flatten the curve. The outcome of this debate, though not drawn to a conclusion, seems to be tilting towards the lockdown approach, with the vast majority of countries opting for this approach. The UK government, having initially explored the herd immunity approach, came down on the fence of the lockdown approach too by late March 2020. Another country, Sweden, adopted the herd immunity approach, and was the only country among the advanced economies to actually take the herd immunity as the main plank of government policy. The Swedish government's main attention in dealing with the infection is to target high risk groups like the elderly and those in care homes as Sweden has one of the highest populations of elderly people living on their own in Europe. Even though the Swedish government decided not to enter into any lockdown mode, it did advise its people to exercise sensible judgement, by which it means judgement on social distancing and self-isolation, while businesses, shops, restaurants and bars by and large stayed open. Its main policy resembling any lockdown was to stop any gatherings of more than 50 people. It is too early to pass an opinion if the Swedish way is better. But the higher number of death tolls in Sweden, which did not have a lockdown approach, when compared with that of Norway, which did have a lockdown approach, suggested that a less restrictive approach may not be the right course of action. Furthermore, by early June 2020, it has been reported that Sweden had the highest mortality rate per capita than the rest of Europe. This did put some intense pressure on the Swedish government as to whether adopting a less restrictive policy as they did in handling the crisis might have been the wrong approach. The protagonists among the Swedish epidemiologists and scientists argued that the overall mortality in the long run may be lower once herd immunity kicks in. The big unknown for this is that one does not know, with any degree of certainty, how long it will take for the herd immunity to reach the 60%-70% threshold. The only advantage of the Swedish model was that it will be easier for life to return to normal, since the measures it took were not that markedly different from before the crisis. However, our concept of normality after Covid-19 may be hard to define. With a lockdown approach, the control may be quicker but there will have to be an unlock plan too. It was easier to execute a lockdown plan and much harder to unlock the plan. The Swedish model can arguably offer an easier exit plan.

Depending on which angle one is looking at the problem from, both schools of thoughts are correct, and they do not have to be mutually exclusive. Indeed, they should be and can be mutually inclusive depending on what stage the pandemic is at. My own view is that the herd immunity approach, while it may have some scientific merits, does not have enough social merits, at least for now. In the modern world, travelling in all forms is a standard and not an exception. People are expected to travel. The modes of transport, such as by rails, ships and airlines are all based on the expectations that travelling is part of modern day life. We all are in a world of fast global travels of such efficiency and convenience that it would be as difficult, if not impossible, to define the meaning of a herd in any country or society. Does herd mean local indigenous population or does it apply to those newcomers too? For a giant modern metropolis like New York City, Beijing or London, is the herd defined by national borders, residency status or passport nationalities? The implementation of such policy, therefore, despite its scientific rationale and the sound principle of having one's own immunity to fight off the virus, must involve a political decision on how herd is defined, requiring very detailed mathematical modelling and detailed plan of execution. So, in order to truly develop the immunity of the herd, the national governments and the global communities have to agree on a broad and general international consensus on what herd in modern day means. Furthermore, a herd immunity here is predicated on a normal and natural immunity of any individual to neutralize a virus and, with so much unknown about Covid-19, this may be a wishful thinking for now, especially as not even the best epidemiologists or scientists can come up with a modelling to best guess how long it will take for herd immunity to reach at least 60% of the population, while the collateral damage to the public may be unquantifiable. Currently, the best guess is that after six months, the herd immunity is less than 10% of the population. Natural immunity, as the words suggest, cannot be rushed, cannot be programmed and certainly cannot be manufactured. Vaccine is the only way to help immunity but even that would take time to develop. It is for these uncertainties that the herd immunity idea was abandoned by the UK after its initial policy debates.

While the lockdown approach has become the standard fire-fighting measure in most countries, and therefore it represented a commonality among countries, the exit plan may have to be different for different countries and cities. A modern giant metropolis full of high-rise buildings with high population density may need a different exit plan to rural villages of scanty population. For instance, London was in the earlier stages of the outbreak the most severely affected city in the UK in April 2020, yet as the crisis passed its peak, there was evidence in May 2020 that London was the first city in the UK where the outbreak came under control. While the other cities in the UK were lagging behind London, it was already suggested that London should be unlocked sooner than the rest of the UK, using a phased approach to unlock the cities in various parts of the country as more regional data became available. And as data on contact tracing and population surveillance are more advanced and specific, a targeted approach can be employed for any lockdown. Such regional lockdown policy was both demonstrably effective and well accepted by the public as witnessed in Beijing in China in the middle of June 2020 due to a cluster of cases and similarly in Leicester in the UK in early July 2020. By the same token, each country may differ in its exit approach. At the end of May 2020, countries like Italy and Spain were beginning to open up by phasing out the lockdown approach. These countries are also opening their borders on the European continent. The civil aviation authority in China also announced that its international and domestic flight schedules would

be significantly scaled up from the lockdown mode
implemented since January 2020.

CHAPTER 5

Advice from the Scientists

It is worth reminding the readers that science has scored some remarkable successes in human endeavours to cope and deal with infectious diseases. Of particular importance is the widespread use of hepatitis B vaccine in the prevention of hepatitis B and the efficacy of its treatment by specific antiviral therapies. Hepatitis B is a specific form of viral hepatitis, transmitted via a non-oral route, usually via needle sharing, sexual contact, childbirth or even blood products contaminated with hepatitis B. This infection can be lethal as it can cause not only liver failure but actually liver cancer, one of the most aggressive cancers known in humans. However, since the introduction of a hepatitis B vaccine for protection against the disease and specific antiviral treatment for its infection, the outlook is now much better. For countries which have already implemented a population-based vaccination programme, the benefits are there for all to see. The incidence of both liver failure and liver cancer has come down; the latter is now regarded as the world's first successful cancer prevention programme by vaccination, a very notable achievement.

The other success is the treatment of HIV infection, a deadly disease first noted in the early 1980s. This infection in the past carried with it not only a huge social stigma as it was first noted in homosexual men, it was also universally known as lethal with patients dying from incurable cancers or fulminating infections as a result of this virus demolishing the immunity system in the patients by destroying the soldiers of our front line of immunity defence called the B lymphocytes. Through the concerted efforts of a large international group of doctors and research scientists, mainly led by the USA, there is now a standard treatment using a combination of specific anti HIV drugs, and which has converted what was previously seen as a lethal disease into what is universally regarded now as a chronic and treatable disease, with manageable treatment related side effects. The principle of the drug treatment is simple and elegant. Basically by using a combination of various antiviral drugs, the virus then has nowhere to hide but be eradicated, achieved by a round the clock presence of these drugs in the body to attack the virus, which then has no chance to remain active to destroy the patient's B lymphocyte. Thus, this will ensure that the patient's immunity will remain intact, so the previous deadly infections which were common in HIV infection, known as opportunistic infections, can be avoided. Opportunistic infections here mean those infections which would only cause problems when the immunity of an individual is compromised.

These two examples are selected here to show that science has now progressed even further since, to a level at which we can actually test to assess objectively how well the treatment is working. For those patients who respond to treatment, the viral DNA will no longer be detectable, thus suggesting control or even eradication of the infection. If the DNA reappears or its level goes up, then it denotes a treatment failure, and in which case other newer and alternative drugs can be used.

However, at its core, science is also about dealing with uncertainties. Our intellectual desire and natural curiosity will help to move us from an uncertain arena to a more certain arena. This is the main driver for the pursuit of science. It all starts with a quest to know the truth, the whats and the hows, which in the beginning can appear to be confusing, speculative and even contradictory. It may even mean different things to different inquisitive minds.

This is the beauty of science. It opens up our imagination and yet disciplines us with the logical thinking through the use of scientific data to prove or disprove a theory. It is only through a painstaking process of laboratory results, real life observations, and proper data validation, again and again by different investigators in different institutions, can the truth be found. This process of converting uncertainties to near certainties always takes a long time, involving real human imagination and experimentation.

The best way to illustrate the painstaking process of scientific achievement is that of Einstein's Theory of Relativity published in 1905. Einstein's theory of general relativity is a cornerstone of modern physics and cosmology. When it was first published, however, there was little hard evidence to show that it was actually correct. It wasn't until 1919, nearly a decade after Einstein began working on the theory, that the British astronomer and scientist Arthur Eddington finally delivered that evidence for this groundbreaking theory with an expedition to the west coast of Africa during a solar eclipse to assess its effect on light.

According to Einstein's theory, light travelling past a massive object like the sun would bend due to the object's immense gravity. With the sun's light blocked out, Eddington measured the positions of distant stars made visible in the background. He showed that when the light from those stars passed by the sun, due to the bending of light by the gravity exerted by the sun, these stars appeared to be in a slightly different place compared to when the sun was not in eclipse. The findings demonstrated that the conception of gravity laid out in the theory of relatively had been correct.

Furthermore, it turned out that the result of his measurements of this deflection was almost perfectly in line with the prediction based on Einstein's formula. This confirmed that light can be bent under the influence of gravity as it passes round the edge of the sun during a total solar eclipse to reach the earth. This wait lasted for about 14 years.

There is another breakthrough which was slightly different but equally illuminating on the nature of scientific discoveries when Watson and Crick proposed the double helix model of DNA at Cambridge University in 1953. Prior to that, it had long been suspected for quite a few years through the study of protein chemistry and X-ray crystallography (which was based on the study of diffraction patterns of X-ray through crystals) that DNA (deoxyribonucleic acid) was quite possibly the foundation of life, based on a collection of building blocks but the exact mechanism still proved elusive. Watson and Crick worked out a double helix model of the DNA, in which each base unit on one of the spiral helix has a fixed counterpart in the other spiral helix, and these two complementary units will form a base pair. This beautiful model became the well-known elegant zipping and unzipping model of DNA and its replications, thus laying the true foundation of life, commonly known as the genetic code. The zipping and unzipping of the double helix is how the whole genetic code folds and unfolds, while passing down the generations. Modifications of this genetic code is by a mutation of the base unit but the function of the double helix as the genetic code is unchanged, and its ability to pass information down the generations remains the same.

The above two examples were used here not because they have entered the realms of popular science folklore known to many people all over the world, but more importantly, to show what science can do. Careful collection of data from precisely carried out experiments need to be meticulously interpreted, topped up with moments of real imagination and brilliance. However, it is equally important to be aware that these were the exceptions and not the rules. Many scientific theories take time to be proved right and more often the theories are proved wrong, or initially proved right only to be proved wrong at a later stage by others. In the pursuit of scientific truth, the competition is fierce, intense, ruthless and yet intellectually enriching.

So, faced with the global challenges of Covid-19,

we need to support and even rely on science to provide for us a leading light in a storm, to give us a pointer in the direction we need to go. Science is the absolute key here. Yet, it is important to be patient. Science cannot be rushed and cutting corners to get fast results is not proper science. Rushing science to come up with the answer would threaten the integrity of science. It is reckless and irresponsible. The public and the politicians must be made aware of this. For Covid-19, the science here is in dealing with human lives so it must be first rate; there is no place for second rate or third rate science, which would only delay or misdirect the progress. It would need real rigour, objectivity and discipline in the uncompromising pursuit of truth, or else the truth is not worth having.

One of the most disconcerting feelings for me as a member of the public going through and witnessing the handling of this crisis was when I heard the leaders and politicians saying, almost as a rhetoric, that they would formulate policies on the basis of scientific and experts' advice. Expert advice I would accept as it reflects an extensive range of expertise and experience achieved over many years on specific areas. Yet I cannot help feeling somewhat uncomfortable when the politicians overuse the word science. So much is yet to be known about Covid-19 scientifically that politicians, in deciding on the policies, may fall into the trap of overreliance on science when science is not ready to be totally relied on. It almost gives out the feeling that they are hiding behind science and may even blame science if the right result is not forthcoming. There is therefore a need for a reality check. Politicians must make decisions based on advice and most up-to-date information but not overplay the promise of what science can bring in the timeframe that the politicians want. Science is apolitical. It needs to be supported, encouraged, funded but never pushed. The examples I quoted above on hepatitis B and HIV have a great and desired outcome because they involved many years of painstaking research studies in the laboratories, in the wards, in the consultation rooms and many more international conferences where there were fierce and vigorous debates on laboratory and clinical data. During that long, arduous and sometimes even dispiriting process of scientific research, there were many false dawns too. This is the real nature of science.

That being said, I do feel optimistic about the eventual outcome and success. Having witnessed the spread of this Covid-19 so rapidly into a global crisis with such a social and economic impact of apocalyptic scale, there is now also a great determination by the international scientific community to pool their efforts, scientific resources, information and data together to deal with this crisis. These scientists do it willingly, under no political influence, nor consideration of any national boundaries. There will be extensive studies on the genomics of the virus, both in mammals and birds, and how the mode of transmission from animals to humans occurs. There will also be huge work involved to see if this virus has different strains with different effects on humans or if any new mutated strains are pathogenically different in causing diseases in the human. All these efforts, joined up globally, will help us to acquire the necessary knowledge in dealing with this virus, especially on the development of a vaccine. Already there are clinical trials scheduled to start in the later part of 2020. And as we know more about Covid-19 through science and epidemiology, we can hope that each wave of Covid-19 is likely to become less severe and even predictable in the timing of its arrival. We would know more about its transmissibility, infectivity and prevalence. These will help us to have an effective and timely contact tracing programme every time a new infection is identified. We will also know more of its pathogenicity, its targeted organs of damage, and the precise mechanism in which cellular damage is done. This information so obtained can be translated to an understanding of the clinical spectrum of the disease, and how the capacity of the body's immunity can be harnessed to mount an immunity response. Treatments can then be designed and vaccines can be produced.

One key area of real human value is to study how

the fruits of successful clinical trials of treatments and vaccines can be harnessed to help the patients in both rich and poor nations. The global community needs to make sure that when an effective and safe vaccine is developed, it is ready for mass production to meet demands in an affordable manner. Equally, a specific antiviral drug or combination of drugs should also be affordable by most to treat those infected. We also need to be sure when is the best time to start treating the infection and how to handle the asymptomatic cases. The studies may be many, though answers can be few. Nonetheless the important answers will be there for us. With all the vast and collective efforts that the global community has put into these various areas, I remain hopeful that science will be pivotal in giving us the answers and help to deliver us to a safer world.

CHAPTER 6

The Social Debate

History has shown that whenever there was a global
crisis, people in general did not change their behaviour in
any significant way when the crisis was over, though the
recovery back to normal may take some time. The recovery
process after an economic crisis may be different from a
post-war situation. There were the expected short-term
adjustments in times of crisis but in the recovery process,
by and large, the behaviour of people is more likely to
reflect their cultural, religious, educational and even ethnic
backgrounds. This diversity is what makes the world so
interesting. We are all used to and welcome this diversity.
This culture of fusion adds colour to our lives and enables
us to appreciate others with different backgrounds. It also
prevents us from being boxed in as stereotypes. There

are no standards, and it is the rich tapestry of fabrics of different colours which makes life exciting and fun.

This time round, with Covid-19, things may be distinctly different and the differences may have a long lasting impact. This is because Covid-19 is such a transformative event. Never before had so many countries imposed almost a total lockdown within such a short timeframe. As a result, there is now already a new discussion among the wider public on what the behaviour psychiatrists would say of how things may change and in the process, how our behaviour may change too.

These changes, from whatever angle one looks at them, stem from a core acceptance that Covid-19 compelled nearly all countries to opt for the lockdown mode for at least six to eight weeks, if not more, and also closed the borders too, in seas, land and air transport. A previously interconnected world by easy and accessible means such as air travel was turned into an inter-disconnected world where travelling is not only difficult, but may even be forbidden or impossible. This lockdown approach was so drastic and groundbreaking that at times it was regarded by some as too draconian and too severe for people to cope with, and too heavy an economical price to pay. International flights were reduced by more than 90%. Many actually see this as the only effective way in flattening the curve of the Covid-19 outbreak. It had to be

as comprehensive as it was brave; there could not be any
loopholes. This is why the initial approach in China in
locking down the city of Wuhan, then the whole province
of Hubei, won such admiration from most other countries.
If you stop people from coming in and going out, then
this virus cannot travel far. Cities and countries do not
welcome visitors for one obvious reason: they don't want
people to bring the virus in. So, exit is desirable, but entry
is unwelcome and must be deterred. There was evidence
that in some countries, notably Singapore, that, having
had initial success in reducing the spread of the infection
by flattening the curve, experienced a second peak almost
entirely due to the arrivals of newcomers, which might
act as the seeding source of another cluster of infection.
Singapore is unique in this as the country depends quite
heavily on immigrants, mainly from South Asian countries,
for much of its infrastructure work. These immigrants were
generally housed in very densely packed small dwellings
which provided fertile grounds for the virus to spread.
The same resurgence of new cases also happened in Hong
Kong in July 2020, when, over a period of three weeks,
Hong Kong experienced a surge of 1,669 cases, making the
total number of cases in Hong Kong since the pandemic
to more than 3,000 (with 15 Covid-19 related deaths). This
figure was higher than the number of cases of SARS Hong
Kong had in 2003. Yet in the early phase of the outbreak,

Hong Kong was riding the storm relatively well with seven deaths in total by the end of June. The reasons were partly due to lessening up of social distancing measures and also the exemption of the 14 days of mandatory quarantine for visitors to Hong Kong such as senior business executives, air crew and seamen. This is seen as the third wave of the Covid-19 attack in Hong Kong, resulting in even more stringent measures imposed by the Hong Kong SAR government. The experience in the severity of the third wave of infection should serve as a reminder to the global community that waves of infection will recur. There are already signs in July of the emergence of a second wave of infection in Europe in countries like Spain and Germany, while the USA has not quite passed its first wave in July. So it once again confirmed that vigilance must be maintained at all times, and the virus will attack where it can, and when it can.

Just as important as lockdown for a country or a city is the importance of social distancing and self-isolation for individuals or a family unit in protecting themselves from infection. So we all are compartmentalized in small units of isolation. The only ways we can connect with the outside world are through the radio, TV, streaming and social media. We all know that the virus spreads by droplets and the droplets cannot travel far. Even if a person carrying the virus sneezes, it travels no more than 1.5 to 2 metres before it falls to the ground and is rendered non-infective. In the face of acute worldwide shortage of personal protective equipment (PPE), gowns, masks, goggles and caps, the use of which all have to be disposable after initial use, the only sure way, which was advised by all countries, to protect oneself from infection is by social distancing and self-isolation. I infect no one and no one infects me, thus hopefully the R value will come down. This distancing means only physical distance so one can still keep in touch with friends and families through telephone or other mobile devices, but one cannot let their grandchildren visit them and give them a hug. The parcel delivery man will ring your doorbell, leave the parcel on your doorstep, and then he would walk away for you to pick up the parcel.

It is the combination of lockdown and social distancing that would change our behaviour, socially, domestically and perhaps even habitually.

For example, in China, the means of enforcing isolation was impressive. In general, nearly all urban cities in China have densely populated housing estates with multiple blocks of high-rise buildings. I have witnessed at first-hand how they dealt with it and how effective it was. There was a designated area where the delivery man simply dropped the parcels and groceries which the residents ordered online. All these orders were labelled with a specific QR code. The estate's security guard would keep an eye on this area and only registered and known residents were allowed to go into this communal area where they could use their smartphones to scan and take the goods which they had ordered. For those who were physically unable to do so, there would be registered volunteers to do it for them. This system worked efficiently and smoothly. There was no theft. It actually enhanced the communal spirit in the housing estate with residents helping one another in times of need, while social distancing was strictly enforced all the time. Small inconveniences were tolerated willingly and welcomed in exchange for safety from acquiring or passing the infection.

Self-isolation is just as important too. Both social distancing and self-isolation are clearly measures which can be taken actively by individuals or family units. The public needed no persuasion. Take the city of Hong Kong as an example. Just like the rest of China, because masks and tests were readily available, and most hospitals had the capacity to cope, the Hong Kong government did not have to impose strict lockdown for the whole city, yet the outcome was still amazingly good, with seven deaths in a population of 7.5 million up to the end of June 2020. Regrettably, such good work was undone by the onslaught of the third wave in Hong Kong in July as a result of opening up of public places, restaurants and lowering of personal vigilance. Some countries had difficulties in implementing social distancing in the beginning. One reason for the slow take up rate of these measures in these countries, mostly in the West, was the misplaced perception among the public that the outbreak was happening so far away that it would not come to them. Then they realized, some weeks later, and all of a sudden, that the wave had arrived, hitting them with a force that shook them all to the core, despite the earlier and repeated warnings from the WHO and the epidemiologists. Initially, there was also individual complacency with the attitude that 'it is not happening to me and it won't happen to me'! These people paid no regard to the social distancing rules and even flaunted in public their somewhat macho disregard. However, once such blatant disregards for public safety were captured by smartphones and uploaded onto the social media, there was a public backlash and outcry against such behaviours. The result was that these disregards rapidly disappeared, and everybody fell in line. This was what peer pressure and public shaming on social media could do, which the police may not be resourced enough to do.

Sandwiched between the lockdown of a city and the practice of social distancing by the individuals, there was the question about what to do with retail shops and leisure industries such as cinemas, restaurants, gymnasiums. Most countries followed what China did earlier in this pandemic when nearly all restaurants, shops, gymnasiums, cinemas and schools were closed. Only essential services were allowed but even these were discouraged. I remember that on the first Saturday I had during the peak of the crisis in China, I walked from my hospital to the subway train station only to find there was hardly anyone in the station. Not only that, there was barely any other traffic on the roads, which on any given Saturday are usually congested with cars and taxis. Outside my hospital there was a long line of waiting taxis, all looking for customers. Many of my colleagues, instead of taking the subway, chose to take taxis to minimize their possible exposure. Many countries had since adopted the same measures as initially implemented in China. In the UK, one of the key indicators that was relayed to the public on a daily basis was the road traffic motoring activity and the use of subways as a guide to the movement of the public to test the compliance of the social distancing and self-isolation advice. This combination of lockdown, closing of non-essential services and social distancing, painful and inconvenient as they were, undoubtedly worked. By the time I left China in the middle of March 2020, the crisis in China had passed its peak and things gradually started to return to normal. I came back to the UK just before the UK entered its peak when all similar measures were introduced, and after six weeks, there were also clear signs that the UK had begun to pass its peak.

As it is now clearly proven that these measures are effective, they are likely to become standard practice for the future in response to the next wave. The public needs no further convincing. This Covid-19 outbreak has given the public an experience and a personal code of conduct on health matters that they are unlikely to forget or forgo. Just like the people in Southern China, especially those in Hong Kong, would not forget the trauma of SARS in 2003 and the public from the Middle East countries would remember the trauma from MERS in 2012, the public of the present global communities would be better prepared for the next wave when it comes.

Clearly one has to be aware of the problems of this social distancing and self-isolation, not to mention the huge and almost immeasurable economic cost. There will always be vulnerable groups in this, and these groups deserve our attention and help. The lonely old men and women in their 70s or 80s living alone whose mobility may be limited and cannot shop freely. The young families with young children who cannot go to school, and live in a small flat or house with limited space, where children are advised not to go out and play with their neighbours. The lack of personal space will cause domestic pressure. It is already quite clear in the UK that domestic violence incidents have risen, with some estimates showing an increase as high as 30%. And the single parent scenario may be even worse in terms of the hardship within the families. The lowly paid group whose living conditions are poor and crowded. The difficulties these people face must not be forgotten and if nothing is done to help them, and the plight they are in is not appreciated by society, then their stress levels will continue to get higher, with each passing day of social distancing and isolation, until some people fail to cope and have a breakdown. Behaviour scientists and psychiatrists are already warning us of such problems and these problems again are universal in nature, no country is exempted. Lives are at stake here, but equally livelihoods are also at stake.

Community help and restoration to normality are clearly desirable but what is the definition of normal, in the face of such a viral attack which we know may come back again? Survey after survey are already showing that people are prepared to socialize less even if the outbreak comes under control. Their shopping and socializing habits such as eating out will be different from before Covid-19. In short, people not only will be making changes in their lifestyle, but quite possibly these changes may be permanent. These are not adjustments in times of difficulties but actual changes, called the New Normal. This will be discussed further in a later chapter.

Another significant change which goes with social distancing is the emergence of a new phenomenon called working from home. This usually refers to people who

normally have worked, prior to Covid-19, the standard
office hours in an office but it can equally apply to those
whose work was less restricted and regimented, such
as those in the creative industries or journalism. The
advantages here are not only to enable social distancing to
reduce cross infections in the congested public transport
systems such as subways or buses during the office rush
hours. Most governments were active in either enforcing or
advising working from home. Just like social distancing, it
does not mean social disconnection. Working from home,
when there is no one to spot check, does not guarantee
the same level of work output but it does allow some
flexibility in the performance of the individual. So, there
is an element of trust here, but it does play a key part in
reducing cross infection. This is a necessary and sensible
trade-off between public health and the productivity of
the individual, though there is so far no study to show that
the productivity is compromised when one is working
from home. The effort in this in most countries was led
by the governments and governments enforced this by
setting their own example. All the people who work for
the government (the civil service) were told to work from
home. This was practised in China and latterly in the UK
and many other countries too. And even when things start
to recover, it is highly likely that the back to the office
plan will be a phased programme by dividing staff into

rotating teams to go to work. For some in the creative industries such as graphic designers, editors, writers and commentators, working from home may even be a much better choice. For instance, I can choose to write this section at a time when it is convenient for me as long as I have my laptop and my Wi-Fi, free from any distraction. If there is noisy building work around me during the day, I can choose to write in the evening when it is quiet, for as long as I can meet the deadline. So by working from home, there are arguably longer but more flexible working hours, which can enhance the creativity and productivity rather than hinder it. Creativity depends on inspiration and not on fixed office hours. For collaboration among the professionals, those in the creative industries will just as easily find another colleague who is equally flexible in engaging with each other outside office hours. One observation to be made was that even the reporters in the media had changed their way of reporting news. These days, every time you see them interview someone, it was never face-to-face in the TV studio but was done either in the open air, with both interviewer and interviewee at least two meters apart using a modified microphone with long arm in between, or if the interview is held indoors, then it will be done using video conferencing facilities such as Zoom.

Overall, therefore, these enforced and obligatory

changes of social behaviour, advised or imposed by governments, to protect ourselves and others from infection with Covid-19 have been very positively received by the public as the benefits were self-evidently clear. The debate here is whether these changes are sustainable when things begin to return to normal and countries start to fire up the economic engine. In my own view, at least some changes are likely to stay in the future. In fact, this is not dissimilar to us as doctors advising our patients that adjustments in lifestyle are necessary in the face of lifestyle diseases, such as obesity, hypertension, and coronary heart disease. We improve our health or prevent chronic diseases by changing our lifestyle in smoking less, exercising more, eating less salty and fatty food, and aided by modern drug treatments where necessary. Over time, our health can then hopefully be improved.

CHAPTER 7

The Cultural Debate on the Use of Masks

Strangely, if there is one issue which caused significant anxiety, debate and uncertainties currently, and which reflected the difference in cultures and people's behaviours between East and West, it would be on the use of surgical masks. The original purpose of surgical masks, as the name suggests, was to protect surgeons when they went into the operating theatre to operate on the patients. In other words, to reduce infection through breathing, as opposed to other masks such as those for cosmetic purposes. Some fictional characters in films such as Darth Vader in Star Wars not only wore masks, he seemed to have a whole set of PPE around him. Others do wear masks too, like the Venetian Masks worn in the annual Carnival of Venice! The latter use of masks is mainly for effect and nothing else. This may also be a cultural phenomenon. In the Islamic culture, it is required for women to wear facial coverings called the burka, though not as intended as masks in the traditional sense of either cosmetic or infection control purposes.

Having spent six weeks in Shenzhen during the most trying time in China and then going through an equally trying time in the UK, I cannot help but notice the difference in attitude between the East and the West. This difference can best be explained on the basis of a difference in the perceived benefits of the use of masks.

The use of masks for the protection from air pollution and droplet infections has always been accepted as a norm for the daily lives of the people in some Asian countries such as China, Japan, Singapore and South Korea. Following the lessons learned in the outbreak of SARS in 2003, from which the public is deeply scarred, the use of masks for personal protection has become habitual and even serves as a sign of good practice. The public in these countries, in times of any viral outbreak, are distinctly praiseworthy and noticeable by how compliant they are in wearing masks and how universal this practice is. Wherever you go and whoever you meet, people are wearing masks in these times. In fact, you will get a strange look from the others if you don't use one. So, in short, the need and the use of masks in times of an outbreak are the social norm, acceptable and practised by all in countries like China, Japan, Singapore and South Korea.

Before I went back to Shenzhen in early February 2020, I had to search for some masks in the UK, with great difficulty, prior to my trip. I even got a strange look when I asked various chemists or supermarkets in the UK if they sold any masks! I knew I had to protect myself and others in doing my work in Shenzhen. In the beginning, masks were in short supply even in China too and our hospital had to ration their use so no one was found wanting. At the peak of the shortage, our staff even worked voluntarily over the weekends and evenings to produce self-made masks and protective shields. When I went to see them in their work room working diligently away one Friday evening, I was profoundly moved. It reflected such a determined and positive attitude on their part in working out one's own solution. None of the staff was an engineer, nurse or even doctor by background, they simply learned all about protective masks and the technical specifications required through the internet. Whether their end product was truly protective was another matter. What matters here was it sent out an unambiguous signal on their reliance on self-sufficiency and willingness in coming up with a solution to produce, however a limited number of masks it may be, to help their colleagues in the hospital. Some masks they made even came with a protective shield.

Yet, I also remembered very clearly, when I was departing for the UK on March 16, 2020, that, apart from those of us of Asian ethnicity, no other passengers in any departure gates in the Hong Kong International Airport were wearing any masks despite the HKSAR governmental advice. This advice was clearly ignored by the non-Asians. I could hardly believe what I saw, as if this international airport was divided into two camps. All the Asians were wearing masks while the non-Asians weren't, strolling about in a nonchalant, carefree manner that one could only admire or ridicule. I actually asked one of the staff why these people were not told to wear masks and their reply to me was that the staff did tell them but none of them took any notice, gesturing that it was of no proven benefits. There was nothing anyone could do as they all had their boarding passes. The difference in attitude was even more obvious when I got back to the UK which was, by then, already heading for a lockdown mode. Only a handful of the British people in public wore masks and the UK government, in issuing their advice, did not advise the public to wear masks throughout the whole period. To be fair, even the WHO did not advocate the widespread use of masks until early June 2020. Before then, it only advised that masks should be worn by those who have symptoms or those involve in patients' care.

So, should masks be used at times like this? As the

immortal line in the Shakespeare play *Hamlet* said: To be or not to be, that is the question! My view is that wearing a mask serves three main purposes. First, to protect one from spreading germs to others if one sneezes or coughs. The second one is not dissimilar to the first one, and that is, to make sure others have less chance of passing germs to us. So, by wearing a mask, the protection works both ways. Let us ask ourselves one question. For example, would we be comfortable if we are stuck in a lift or a plane, and the chap next to us keeps coughing or sneezing without a mask? The answer is indisputably obvious. The third reason is symbolic but equally important in its significance. It sends out clear messages to all others that we take this protection very seriously. It fosters trust in each other and enhances a sense of civic responsibility. Everyone knows the importance of hand washing. By not wearing a mask, one can be forgiven for inferring that hand washing may not be taken seriously by that someone too. By wearing a mask, it will create the opposite impression. So, this is a signal to others that you are doing your bit to protect them and, therefore, they should also do their bit likewise to protect you.

While the arguments above have not been proven conclusively by medical or epidemiological studies, most countries in the West did not advocate strongly the use of masks at the beginning of the outbreak, though no one advised against it. It was left to the individual to decide. There was this cultural attitude that wearing protective masks in public might be seen as socially odd. Michael Jackson wearing a mask in public certainly would not raise any eyebrows, as he was regarded as a rock idol who set the trend, rather than followed the trend, and as such, any odd practice would be tolerated, if not imitated, by the public. After three months into this pandemic, there was very clear evidence in the West that there was a major shift in the attitude towards the necessity of wearing a mask. Articles and opinions began to be written and published in respectable newspapers in various countries advocating that wearing a mask would be beneficial. The only argument against it, if any, was that it was inconvenient. Another initial argument that was put forward by some, which could be instantly dismissed out of hand, was that it gave the wearers of mask a false sense of security! How could there be a false sense of security when the whole society was surrounded by insecurity? The rationale for this subsequent change of attitude was very simple. If this is good and important for the healthcare workers to protect themselves by wearing masks, why should the public not wear masks? Protecting should be for all and at these times of crisis, there was simply no worthy argument against wearing masks for any cosmetic, social or cultural reasons.

To my own satisfaction, this fundamental difference

between the East and the West has changed and people
are now beginning to accept the necessity of wearing
masks in barely a month after I arrived back in the UK
in March 2020. On March 30, Austria became the first
country in Europe telling people to wear masks when
shopping. The need for this was then adopted in Germany
and France. The WHO was then indicating that it was
actively considering updating its guidelines on the use of
masks. The USA, as of April 2020, started to recommend
the use of masks by the public. It is therefore hard not
to draw the observation that one of the key reasons that
China, Singapore and South Korea were successful in
containing the infection was the general use of masks by
the public, upon which most impartial observers have now
agreed. By the middle of May, when the UK government
was deliberating how best to unlock society, one of the
key messages was that it advised the public to use facial
coverings in public. In France, no passenger without a
mask would be allowed to go on their Metro, while in
London Tube stations, still only about one third of the
passengers were wearing masks. Even the staff working
in the White House for the President of the USA have
now been advised to wear masks. This may be a bitter pill
for the US Administration to swallow as the USA is so
used to being the policymaker and trendsetter in global
issues. The Westernization of this practice from the East,

a practice which was previously thought to be a trivial and dismissible matter, has now been accepted as universally standard advice. So, the debate for masks is now over, the practice is now universally recommended. For the UK government, in its handling of the crisis during the peak, at least it is honest enough to use different words such as facial coverings instead of the word masks, for the very simple reason that the demand for masks cannot possibly be met if this is an official recommendation. Why bother to ire the public when one knows something is not possible? The problem for the supply of masks in the UK was only resolved by June 2020 and as the UK started to open up, the government then announced around the middle of July 2020 that everyone going into a shop should wear a mask in an effort to minimize the early emergence of the second wave. In effect, it means people in public would be asked to wear a mask. Though belated, this advice was necessary as data have shown that in China, 82% of people wear masks in public while in Spain, the figure was 86%. The figure in the UK was paltry at 36%.

The next big challenge, however, having accepted the need and the necessity of wearing masks for infection control, is the very tough problem of ensuring supplies meeting the demands. After all, the making of masks is regarded as a low tech, low skill and low profit margin piece of manufacturing, so the making of such protective

surgical masks in most advanced economies has been
dished out to other countries. This was a major and
acute problem worldwide. At the peak of the crisis, it was
estimated that at least one third of the world's population
were or are in lockdown mode. Assuming even one mask
per person per day is needed, the production targets from
the manufacturer will be staggering – there simply was not
enough manufacturing capacity in any country to satisfy
the demand if the public are all advised to wear mask. Most
of the masks in the world are made in China and countries
in the East. China, Japan and South Korea are self-sufficient
in producing adequate masks for their own people. If,
however, countries in the West advocated the use of masks,
then the supply would simply dry up within days. It was
therefore clear some form of rationing was needed and
that these countries could only restrict the use of masks in
the hospital settings because of the certain knowledge that
any such advice to the public would lead to mass hysteria
and panic in searching for a mask. So, it was prudent not
to advise on the undeliverable and unachievable. By the
middle of May, the manufacturer capacity was catching
up and the debate was finally over. While this debate was
going on before in the West, it is interesting to point out
that in the East, designer type or personalized masks are
already on the market for purchase so one can match the
scarf or the outfit with a coloured mask, patterned mask,

or logo mask, not dissimilar to buying an Apple Watch with a collection of straps of different colours to match the occasion and the outfit. In fact, I have seen newspaper reports on recent fashion shows where the models walked onto the catwalk with masks of different colours and patterns to match the latest fashion. In Paris, long since hailed as the capital of fashion, masks have even been used as a trendy accessory too. So, we can turn the argument upside down by seeing this not only as a health protection measure but also as a personal accessory and expression of trendiness to be used when and where necessary!

CHAPTER 8

The Role of Technology

The first thing to discuss here is the word 'test'. To me,
it is such a generic word that it needs proper explaining.
It can mean different things to different people. There is
considerable debate, sometimes even misunderstandings, in
the international press about tests. The WHO advises that
the key to fighting the virus is to test, test, test. But then,
what do tests actually mean? The main area for heated
debate was on the issue of what does testing for the virus
mean? In general, there are two main types of tests to be
clarified here. The test for the actual presence of the virus
is called the nuclei acid amplification test (NAAT or NAT).
This test is for the detection of the virus in establishing the
diagnosis for both the patients and carriers, which mean
asymptomatic carriers, using a technique called rt-PCR

(reverse transcriptase polymerase chain reaction). This test is vital for contact tracing as well. The best outcome in dealing with the outbreak is to test extensively for the virus in both the patients, contacts and the carriers. This test is a much more technically advanced test as it involves the creation of a primer based on the nuclei acid (either DNA or RNA) sequence of the virus. It involves taking a nasopharyngeal swab or a throat swab. It is also commonly known as the antigen test as it tests for the presence of the virus which carries the antigen. It therefore does not depend on the immunity response of the person being tested. This test is the main test used in China and other countries such as South Korea, Singapore, and Germany. In fact, China is the first country that can carry out this test on a massive scale, with reagents produced by a major Shenzhen biotechnology company called BGI, which was the first in the world to come up with such a NAT test. The other main test is for the presence of antibodies to the virus. This is a test which is being developed both as a blood test and as a point-of-care, finger-pricked test. This is technically much simpler but the detection of antibodies does depend on a normal immune response of the person being tested. Both the test for the virus and the test for the antibodies have their advocates. There is a gap, however, in that the NAT can detect the virus before the body can mount a sufficient immune response to produce the antibodies in sufficient titres to be detectable. So the antibody test is host dependent and there is a window of negativity before the immune response can fully kick in. The other mandatory step for both of these tests, which somehow is not properly discussed in the international press, thus the public not being properly informed, is that for both types of tests to be of value in helping the patients and the public, there must be assurance of the adequacy of supplies of the proper reagents used in these tests. In other words, the tests have to be routinely available, and not intermittently available. The quality and accuracy of these tests are also dependent on the technical know-how in carrying out such tests. So, for both types of tests, the reproducibility, precision and accuracy have to be properly worked out before they are rolled out for routine use. To ensure the quality and the validity of the tests, they also have to be approved and certified by the national licensing authority in each country. In other words, for both the nucleic acid and the antibody tests, there is a strict quality standard to be met to protect the public from getting false information. An erroneous test result can potentially do more damage than no test. Overestimation (false positives) and underestimation (false negatives) must be minimized before such tests, some of which may be commercially marketed as easy to perform by any untrained personnel, can be used for the public. All health agencies have a salient duty to assure the public that these kits are reliable, accurate and informative. The worst outcome is an unreliable test leading to erratic actions or even panic. Countries as advanced as the USA and the UK were finding it extremely difficult to come up with a test of such quality to be used on a massive scale to satisfy the demands of the public, despite both countries boasting about being home to some of the most advanced high-tech biomedical giants. So even when the WHO advised that the key to control of this pandemic is to test, test and test, most countries are unable to do so in such a short period of time because of lack of supply of the necessary reagents and lack of standards of how to ensure uniformity of the test and its results.

Furthermore, there is still a lot of public misconception and confusion, especially around the antibody test. Most people would like to know if they do have the Covid-19 antibodies so that their freedom of movement can be far less restrictive. The difficulty here is the reliability of the test as opposed to its availability and convenience. It is human nature to expect the test to be as convenient as a finger-pricked test like testing for blood sugar for a diabetic patient or a urine pregnancy dip test for a woman suspected of being pregnant. In the case of Covid-19, the reliable tests are based on the traditional blood test, mainly from the Swiss company called Roche and the US companies called Abbot and Ortho Diagnostics, all three being world leaders in the field of diagnostics. They are reliable but not quite available to all, especially since they need a sophisticated piece of expensive equipment to process these tests. The available ones, sometimes marketed as a finger-pricked test, may not be reliable, and are provided by upstarts which may lack the expertise the big pharmaceuticals have acquired over the years. It is questionable whether some of these tests even have a licence. They may be marketed as health products, which have a less stringent regulatory process. And, just like herbal medicines, they may be purchasable off the shelf in a supermarket.

If these logistical problems about supplies, reagents and standards can be resolved, then one can aim for a public health orientated and long-term policy by doing both tests for the diagnosis, contact tracing, population surveillance and assessment of immunity status on the basis of a large epidemiological study to assess the immunity status of the population. This has been done successfully in other viral diseases and the benefits are clearly demonstrated. In hepatitis B for instance, both the antigen and the antibody tests are often done as a combined set of blood tests to give the clinicians better information about a given patient. The ideal finding would be one who is antigen negative but antibody positive, which means that this person is protected by his or her own immunity, having been previously exposed, and can be freed from social isolation.

This first group, in my view, may turn out to be the largest group in any population study. If the result shows antibody negative and antigen positive, then this infection can either be from a symptomatic patient or an asymptomatic carrier (estimated to be affecting up to 25% of infected patients). As such, they should be isolated, and contact tracing initiated. This group can be considered for specific antiviral treatment if available, or enrolment into an ethically approved clinical trial for early pre-emptive interventional treatment by antiviral agents or other means. If the tests show both antibodies and antigen are negative, then this group can be actively considered for immunization by a Covid-19 vaccine. Given the current fast tracked and global race in clinical trials on new, antiviral treatments and the development of a vaccine, it is likely they can be available in less than two years' time.

Another area worthy of special mention is how technology can now help to transform the way medical care is delivered. There are apps already being used in China to check the infection risk for an individual or contact tracing for an infected patient. There are also apps for the identification of hot spots, which are areas of clusters of infection, say, in a shopping mall, so people can avoid going to these areas. In this, China is leading the rest of the world. There are several reasons for this lead. First, China is already technologically very advanced in this new age of the Fourth Industrial Revolution involving artificial intelligence, big data, and supercomputer. Second, the Chinese people are entirely comfortable with the multi functionalities of the smartphone. They are techno savvy. The Chinese people are not only comfortable with the smartphone, but they are actually enthusiastic about the convenience and the usefulness of getting real time information about the infection that the apps on the mobile phone can offer. The smartphone is, without exaggeration or exception, their constant and ever faithful companion. Third, since China was the first to go through the crisis, it had the advantage of being four to six weeks ahead of other countries in developing medical apps for such purposes. Just before I left China in March 2020, my colleagues had already shown me apps on various occasions on where to avoid going. There was a real time demonstration of the state of a city, an area, or a mall. Now these apps are further developed into a more refined system like a traffic light with green for a safe area and red for a no-go area, in a way which is similar to being informed ahead of the road traffic conditions while one is driving. So GPS (Global Positioning System) for a driver to seek the right directions can become another form of GPS (global personal safety) for infection prevention! Now other countries in Europe and the USA are assessing their own IT and smartphone capabilities for the same purposes. The UK government is planning to launch a blue-tooth based track and trace app, jointly developed with Apple and Google, by the end of 2020.

IT has also helped and even revolutionized the way doctors and patients interact. This is now known as telemedicine for consultation. The advantage of this is that the chance of cross infection is zero, as compared with the traditional face-to-face consultation, since it is done via a mobile device for consultation or over a telephone if a verbal consultation is all that is clinically needed. Many hospitals in China have already started this service and indeed, I have also done this in Shenzhen over the last few years, sometimes even in the evenings. It did not give me any extra stress and the patients all appreciated it. In the UK, the GP service also has moved significantly, since the onset of Covid-19, towards the use of telemedicine. Before Covid-19, hospitals and GP practices were nearly always full of patients and it was impossible to keep patients at two metres apart while they were waiting, often measured in hours in the waiting rooms. The doctors were busy, the staff were busy and the patients were kept waiting. So everyone was stressed by a hectic and unwelcoming environment while what is needed for a medical consultation is precisely the opposite such as peace, privacy and convenience. So, by moving towards telemedicine, everyone is safer and for the patients, no travelling is involved. Moreover, and this is the most important aspect, they could wait in the comfort of their own homes. In the last few years, certainly in China, telemedicine was already developing at a very fast pace but as an unintended consequence of Covid-19, the modern advanced economies are all resorting to this form of remote consultation to be the main plank of dealing with the crisis. In the UK, for example, the service provided by the primary care sector has moved almost completely, over the course of three months, from a face-to-face, appointment based system to the use of telemedicine for consultation. In fact, a form of telemedicine was already introduced in the NHS in the UK about seven years ago but this recent change has taken up the scale by several notches. This change was hugely welcome by both the patients for its convenience and by the doctors for its safety and speediness. There was hardly any negative press on this. This practice is now only going to stay and will be further fine-tuned. One can really see how telemedicine and teleconsultation have truly come of age now because of Covid-19. It will become the norm of the healthcare services in the very near future.

On the world stage, a shining example was the most recent G20 meeting hosted by Saudi Arabia in April 2020. It was done by live video conferencing. If the top people in the top 20 countries can get to talk to each other in a real time video scenario, what is there not possible to achieve, when it comes to networking and conferencing? The one hidden advantage, not widely reported in the press, was the huge sigh of relief from the security services in the vast operation that had to be taken to protect, quite apart from Covid-19 infection, the top 20 leaders and their entourage from harm's way. It could also be confidently predicted that none of the top 20 leaders would see it as an opportunity missed. They would much more likely have breathed a sigh of relief for not having to pose for photo shoots and touch of wine glasses as part of the customary diplomatic niceties. It is not suggested for one minute that the formalities of such meetings must be changed. Nevertheless, it is important that at this time of a pandemic, the world leaders not only have to advise the public what to do, but also set an example to follow their own advice. They should do what they preach. There can be no double standards at times like this. Fewer presidential or prime ministerial pomp displays of power and privileges would also be appreciated by the public. Working from home is the same concept applicable to the leaders as to the public. In the case of these leaders, their working from home means they are working in their own countries and not jetting around, while trying to deal with jet lag.

CHAPTER 9

The Economic Challenges

The economic impact of this pandemic was widely thought
to be dire, quite possibly the worst since records began,
and no country could escape from it. This devastating
economic impact, in light of the nature and the severity of
the pandemic, as well as the almost universal lockdown
approach by nearly all countries, was both predictable and
unavoidable. If countries and cities were shut down, how
would there be any economic activities? All the remaining
activities that were evident anywhere at the height of the
crisis were healthcare related services or logistic support
for essential items such as food and groceries. These can
range from the urgent building of new hospitals to the
searching from, competing with, and importing from other
countries in the global markets to block buy masks, PPE,

ventilators, to even asking final year medical students to
help out in the wards or inviting retired doctors and nurses
to return to work. All these would cause huge extra drain
on economic resources. The activities that traditionally
generate economic growth, such as retailing, leisure
services, hospitality services, food and beverage services,
entertainment services and sporting events, were all shut
down. Some international airline carriers cut their flights
by 90%. Nearly all commercial flights, instead of flying
their ways in the sky, were grounded. Instead of having
most planes flying in the sky somewhere over the earth, we
had the debacle of seeing all airports full of planes on the
ground. At the height of the crisis in China and in the UK,
I took some isolated short walks around the city centres
and found they were like ghost towns, with hardly any
activity to be noticed. Even though some shops, apart from
restaurants, in Shenzhen remained open, there was no one
doing the shopping while the lone shop assistants often
were checking things on their mobile phones. In the UK,
shops were all closed, apart from supermarkets. There was
an eerie silence from the complete lack of human activity as
everyone was at home.

Economic growth would head south towards a severe
recession because of the restrictions of movement of people,
goods and services. Lack of human movement also meant
closures of factories as the workers were told to stay home.

This mother of all pandemics was attacking us globally on multiple fronts, and shook our previously unbridled confidence as never before. Investors may not spend to invest and consumers may be too cautious to spend even if the Covid-19 attack recedes. Confidence breeds confidence while pessimism is infectious, just like the virus.

The World Trade Organization (WTO) estimated that global trade could fall by between 13% and 32% in 2020. The Oxford University Economics Centre estimated that the world's GDP will shrink by 7% in the first six months of 2020, doubling that seen in the last global financial crisis in 2008.

Without economic activity, people's livelihoods would suffer. The rich would become less rich, the not so poor will become poor and the poor will become poorer. Those who have had a job to go to would suddenly be told they did not need to turn up for work as there was no work. I found myself learning a new word in English – 'furlough'. I have never seen a word being printed and spoken so much in all the papers and media, that one might even be forgiven in thinking that this was the only word to be used to describe the economic challenges posed by Covid-19. Sadly, I soon realized that it was not a bad word. Indeed it was a very apt word to illustrate the dire economic situation that most of the world was in. If one word can be used to teach the future economic students to appreciate the global effect of Covid-19, it would be this word 'furlough'. Not only was there no work, but even if there was, the government and your employer would have told you: do not turn up for work, we would help you to go on a sort of paid unemployment, the only condition is to stay at home!

Faced with the extraordinary situation of Covid-19, extraordinary economic measures were also necessary to alleviate the threat to livelihoods. Nearly all governments had to accept and deal with the unprecedented economic impact of Covid-19. How else could one stop infection of the masses since there was still so much unknown about the virus, still no effective treatment and no vaccine in sight, apart from the complete and enforced isolation from one person to another? All countries faced the same problems and all countries, quite rightly and in unison, decided that human welfare comes before economic growth, as without humans, there wouldn't be any economic growth. The conventional economic orthodoxy, first introduced in the West and since learned by the East, is that in a capitalist system, it is the market which knows best in how to use private capital to allocate resources and generate prosperity, while governments know next to nothing. The free marketeers ventured that governments only know how to overregulate and generate bureaucracy, which can be detrimental to the creation of prosperity, so their thinking goes. It is better to have a small government which can do only a few things and not get in the way, than a big government which wants to do everything but does it wrong against traditional market orthodoxy. Covid-19 turned that view upside down. In times of national or global crises such as wars or pandemics like Covid-19, people do need a big government. They need the government to take decisive and big actions that no multinationals or individuals can take. So within a short period of six months, a traditional small government model with a market-based approach to the economy and a prudent government budget was replaced by a big government model with a 'whatever it takes' approach. The ambition of making economic growth the cornerstone of policies in any government was turned by Covid-19 into a great convergence of most governments in setting the priority to fight the virus first or lives will be lost. Not surprisingly, as the world passed its peak of the crisis in late May, there were the usual voices from the right wing sector of the political divide in arguing for a quicker re-opening up of the economy despite the outbreak not having reached the end. There were also demands from the left of the political divide in arguing for continuation of lockdown until the crisis was truly over. A balanced approach has to be reached. The public accepted that it was the right thing to do to fight the virus first. It was indeed a no-brainer. Nearly all independent and international based surveys pointed to an overwhelming majority of the public supporting their national governments in their 'whatever it takes' approach. The fight of the virus should drive the economy but not let the economy drive the fight of the virus. All governments, whatever the political ideology, made the right call by spending big money to help, with money they don't have. In other words, issue cheques now and worry about the debt later. Some cheques issued in the USA to help the poor at the height of the crisis apparently had the signature of their present Commander in Chief on the cheque.

Was this throwing money at the problem necessary? Yes it was. Not only was every government doing that, nearly all the world economic pillars of authority like the IMF and OECD supported that too. The human impact of Covid-19 was simply too dire not to do so. Legislative bodies passed the emergency programme of massive cash support with speed and minimal fuss. There was not a single opposing voice. It was as unanimous an action as one could imagine. The action would send out a real message to unite the world in its fight against Covid-19. This was the great convergence, the great consensus.

Many governments made mistakes in the initial stages of the crisis. None of them was flawless. The main criticism being a delay in responding seriously to the outbreak. Nearly all the countries in the West were unprepared and underestimated the risk of Covid-19 from the beginning, despite what had happened in China and the warnings from the WHO. It is always difficult to prepare for a storm especially if the storm comes at such a ferocious speed. This state of unpreparedness, together with the collective complacency of the risk of the crisis by the government and, let it be said, the public too, was the reason why we were where we were. There were not enough masks, not enough PPE, not enough ventilators, not enough ICU beds, and not enough healthcare workers. This not only led the public to panic, but the government to panic too. Logistic chains were disrupted so the supplies, even if available, could not be transported quickly to where they were needed.

The economic measures subsequently undertaken to manage the damage were both mindboggling and comprehensive, but necessary. Most countries now guaranteed the staff salary of the small to medium businesses (some up to 80% of the salary) for three months while on furlough, though capped at a certain level. The UK government has since extended this for four more months till October 2020. Self-employed people were helped in a similar way. Businesses big or small could apply for low interest loans with the government as the guarantor. Banks were encouraged to be active and less strict with their loans rather than the loans requests going through the usual risk assessment process (credit rating). In the case of Covid-19, it was the governments who were encouraging

the banks to be more responsive to their customers than
to their shareholders. For those few big businesses such as
the big banks, which were still making profits, they were
told not to pay dividends to the shareholders. The needs
of the global economy in helping to manage the crisis
were put before paying dividends to the global and big
institutional investors. These firefights initially scared off
the stock markets all over the world. The bigger the stock
markets, the heavier the fall, because that was where all
the money was invested or gambled with. They feared a
complete meltdown, and even feared the end of capitalism.
The markets, managed and monitored by all the hedge
fund geniuses, armed with pre-programmed sell and buy
orders of slide rule precisions, backed up by sophisticated
mathematical models, did not anticipate the arrival of
this RNA. It was hard to bet against a counterparty which
did not know how to play the game. But, to the credit
of coordinated central banks and government actions
in most countries, the stock market's fall became much
more manageable by late May 2020. Fear of financial
collapse was allayed. The initial over-reaction and panic
then calmed down. The lack of debate or even political
opposition to the governmental actions also indicated
clearly that the vast majority of the public, and the wealthy
few, all shared the same views. The cataclysmic event
compelled all of us to think of and help each other. It was

the first pandemic that all of us face in our generation, and is the most severe global pandemic in the last 100 years. History will judge us solely by how we responded to this crisis. None of the press would opine that these economic policies were wrong. Covid-19 is an act of nature. It would be so wrong, untimely and selfish to start a debate purely to score political or economic points based on ideological backgrounds.

Let us now see if we can look into the near future and see what might then be the debates.

It was commonly assumed that Covid-19 would recede by the summer and so the lockdown might be less restrictive with a phased, risk assessed approach for a gradual unlocking process. The lockdown came quite suddenly because of the urgency of dealing with the crisis, but then the reversal of the lockdown must be done carefully to avoid a second wave being rekindled due to significant residual cases, the detection of which is still woefully inadequate especially when many imported cases from abroad were starting to appear, as happened in Singapore in May 2020 and Hong Kong in July 2020. In the best-case scenario, the control of Covid-19 would be moving in the right direction in the second half of 2020. That being so, the economy should also start to recover. Cautious economists and pragmatists warned that we should not expect a quick rebound in the economy. The overall growth for the economy may just make it into a positive territory but nowhere near at the pace which some would hope for. The economy does not work like the stock market whose up and down swings are driven mainly by greed and fear. It certainly cannot be switched off and then on, like a light switch. Furthermore, this slow recovery may be such that there will be no immediate gain in the real economy in areas such as employment rate, consumer spending or growth in service industries. The supply chains may also not recover fast enough after such disruption and indeed, some suppliers would have gone out of business by the time the real economy starts to recover. By real economy, it is meant as an economy not sustained by spending from the government. Just like a person recovering from a major life saving surgery, he would not be advised by his doctor to start going back to work straight away, as he will need time to adjust and recuperate to his full fitness. The economy needs to recuperate first too before it can run along at full throttle.

There is also bound to be some major rethink and questions on another real global issue and that is the role of globalization. Will there be a need to upgrade globalization to version 2? The version 1 of globalization has served the world well and nearly all countries enjoyed economic growth from it. China is a case in point. It grew so well that it is now the second largest economy in the world.

The main reason for its growth was because it became the Factory of the World, backed up by all the associated and necessary advantages which China can offer, such as a supply of skilled and cheap labour force which few countries can match. Capital investments were poured into China. Foreign direct investment, mostly through Hong Kong initially, was able to help China to develop a very strong manufacturing base with modern know-how, modern supply chains, and modern sourcing of materials and components, aided by the add-on values provided by the famed resourcefulness, hard work ethics and industriousness of the Chinese people. All these helped to transform China from primarily a rural, agricultural-based economy historically into a modern manufacturing giant with a very strong industrial base. At the same time, while China was growing economically, uninterrupted over the last four decades to climb up to the G2 position, other advanced economies chose to move up the value chain and as a consequence, vacated and then outsourced their manufacturing capacity, and in so doing, gradually lost their manufacturing base, which they had acquired since the First Industrial Revolution, to other countries known as the emerging markets of the Third World. The production of non-trendy, low margin products such as electronics, clothing, toys, medical supplies and non-generic drugs were transferred out, especially to China, which soaked them up as a giant engine for economic growth. In time, the manufacturing base of the advanced economies began to get weakened and even ignored. They only looked up the value chain and never looked down and, even if they did look down, they could only see things which they knew they could buy cheaply, easily and in bulk from abroad. There is nothing to be concerned about, so they thought, as the efficiency in logistics and the supply chains would see to it that they would not be found wanting. Let all these products from China all go to places like Walmart. After all, Walmart is an American company, not a Chinese company – and then Covid-19 struck.

The fallacy and the risk of this type of thinking has really been exposed by this pandemic when nearly everyone from everywhere wanted nearly the same things. Questions are being asked. Have the advanced economies in the West, in endorsing globalization of trades, been up there at the top of the value chain for so long that they have forgotten the most basics of know-how? They have achieved the high-tech expansion at the expense of losing home-based manufacturing capabilities. Have they used their brains so much in designing chips and algorithms in setting the trend for the future that they forgot how to work the machine to make ordinary but essential products? One thing that was so obvious for all to see was that the advanced economies were even fighting one another for the supplies of masks and PPE. Who would ever imagine or contemplate a scenario, say, in January 2020, that the richest countries in the world would find it harder to procure masks, PPE and ventilators than microchips? The scenario was not even in the script. As a consequence, the public could not protect themselves with masks, the medical and nursing staff did not have enough PPE. Hospital staff were scared and governments started to panic. There was even the spectacle of a planeload of masks from China landing at an US airport – and who would have imagined that such an ordinary air freight would make the headlines! The Chinese public may feel proud and delighted they were helping the USA, while the American public may feel the opposite, that their pride had been dented and the Chinese were showboating; the contrast in perception could not have been more different. The fact remained the same, but the interpretation could be entirely the opposite. It reminded me of a line from Shakespeare's play *Richard the Third*: A horse, a horse, my kingdom for a horse!

I am mindful that years ago, during the height of the oil embargo by the Arab nations in 1973, the US Department of Energy then built a strategic oil reserve to meet the oil demands of the USA for at least 90 days. This was a sound and wise move. It reassured the public, just in case things got worse with the oil embargo.

Perhaps globalization is so successful and the just-in-time delivery motto is working so well, so smooth that no one would contemplate the need for a major review of the definition of essential items which may demand a similar approach to that of the strategic oil reserve designed 50 years ago in the 1970s. The world has since seen various viral attacks from SARS to MERS to Ebola, so essential items should also include those which will be needed in fighting viruses too. There is now a major call for a just-in-case approach in addition to just-in-time. The policy planners over the years did not feel there was a need for such a move as globalization links up countries and economies in such an interdependent way. But the just-in-time motto puts too much emphasis on efficiency without due regard that it sacrifices resilience. Nearly all advanced economies, with perhaps China as the only exception, suffered the consequences of lack of manufacturing resilience or had a vision for a viable stockpile of, say 30 days, of essential items such as masks, PPE or ventilators. Now all that conventional wisdom has to be unlearned and discarded as a result of Covid-19. The painful experience of Covid-19 showed clearly that there is a need to re-look at ways to differentiate essential items and non-essential items. For the essential ones, home-grown capacity must be available or at least at short notice. This would require manufacturing nimbleness. China, from my own experience in early February 2020, right after the two weeks national holiday of Spring Festival, went through the same problems with acute shortage of PPE and masks. However, the manufacturing prowess of China is such that, despite the fact that factories were closed down for a two-week period for the national holidays, it was rapidly able to catch up to be in self-sufficiency state by late February, and some of these factories were called back early by having their holidays closure curtailed. By late March, not only there were sufficient supplies of such essential items, but China was able to export these to help other countries. Regrettably, what was essentially a goodwill gesture of help and a typical trade transaction between China and some countries that wished to buy such goods from China in difficult times was mischievously and sarcastically labelled by some as the Mask Diplomacy or Diplomacy of Generosity. People were unwillingly to see fair trade for what it is. If I wish to pay someone to paint my house, I will pay him and wish him to make a profit so next time he can provide the same service. In any bilateral transaction, trust in the other party is both an essential and a smart practice.

In addition to the acute problems posed by Covid-19 from December 2019, there were already intense tariff disagreements which began in 2016 when the present US President made an election pledge that he saw tariffs on imports from China as one of the main tools of his 'America

First' campaign. Since then, this had led to an escalation from a trade dispute to a trade war between the USA and China, with a major shift towards protectionism. Covid-19 has given extra impetus to this disagreement. Already there are moves and discussions in some countries wishing to withdraw and relocate factories, mainly those based overseas in China, back to their home countries. In other words, some countries now feel a need to re-establish a home-based, broad-based manufacturing sector so that basic and essential items can be provided in times of need. World trades may have to be reset to come up with a modified form of globalization version 2 perhaps, balancing just-in-time with just-in-case. But, if there is a globalization version 2, the process itself will be arduous and very time consuming. Version 1 sped up the world, Version 2 will slow down the world. This Version 2 may also be incompatible with the current trend of protectionism and tariffs. Before long, a global system that served the trading world so well in the last 40 years will become chaotic, factionalized and most certainly, politicalized. Trade will not be economy driven but politically driven. In this version 2, the world is not flat after all.

But globalization, if truth be told, is not a recent development or invention. It has also been pointed out by some in the academic circles that globalization as we know it now was mainly a Eurocentric model following the discovery of the New World by Christopher Columbus in 1492 and discovery of the sea route from Europe to India by Vasco da Gama in 1497. Europe enjoyed unrivalled success and power as a result of these discoveries. Through conquest and colonization, trade boomed like never before but at the terms dictated by the Europeans. The model then metamorphized after WW2 to the formation of the World Trade Organization (WTO). This, together with the advance of air and sea freights, allowed global trades to boom in every corner of the world. Hence it is called globalization. It was even thought to be so successful that the world has become a level playing field in which everyone has an equal stake. The world is flat, and it is also fair. However, a recent academic book published by Harvard University put forward an interesting idea that historically, globalization started from the year 1000 CE, almost 500 years before Columbus and da Gama. The earth was also flat then, fair trade was done on land mass between Eastern Europe, Western Asia, the Middle East and Far East linking some of the oldest nations in the world at the time. Trade flourished with Venice as the terminus in Europe and Xian in China as the terminus in the East. This is the Silk Road, called because trade in one of the most desirable commodities then was silk. In other words, trade is as ancient as civilization itself and trade has been globalizing all the time by whatever means available at a given time in history. Trade is very much part of the DNA make-up of human endeavours as a tool to increase our prosperity. Trade helped humans to get to know one another, of whatever background, religion and culture, to freshen us up with more exchange of cultures, ideas and goods as trade. Therefore, any major reset of global trade should preferably be based on global needs and not regional needs.

We live now in difficult and testing times. Difficult because of the economic havocs Covid-19 has wreaked on us, testing because the havocs may prompt many countries to rethink the future of globalization and supply chains. How much can we still rely on this model and if so, how reliable is it? Would we be caught short again? Would there be a new globalization model mixed with protectionism and tariff? Should there be a model with an acceptable level of stock control, like the strategic oil reserve in the USA, to cushion us from future shock? These are hugely important questions for all to consider, answers to which will have impact for generations. Policies need to be prepared and discussed, taken into account manufacturer's interests, national interests and international interests. If mishandled, the consequences may be even worse than Covid-19.

CHAPTER 10

Politicization of Covid-19

This is an important, even though it may also be a sensitive or controversial, chapter. Politics, some would say, is the art of the possible. I would add that politics can also reflect the dark art of opportunism, and the acquisition of self-serving interests by attacking your opponents, using irresponsible language and spreading falsehood. Of course, the world cannot function without good politics, whatever the systems of governance tools may be. In general, good politics and bad politics are often noticeable, sometimes even glaringly obvious, and, most of the time, the discerning public can tell the difference.

My own experience of going through Covid-19, initially in China and then in the UK, ought to be shared with the readers.

I was in the UK when it was first brought to the attention of the world that there was a viral outbreak in the city of Wuhan in China. It started in December 2019 and the WHO was notified. I knew by the middle of January 2020, the city of Wuhan was the epicentre and the rest of China was also affected. The suddenness caught everyone by surprise. One of the most important factors to which the Western press did not pay significant attention was the unique timing of the outbreak, coming just before the Spring Festival (Chinese Lunar New Year). It is by far the most important festival in the Chinese calendar and has been for more than 3,000 years in the civilization of China. The significance and the importance attached to it cannot be overemphasized. The Spring Festival lasts for seven days but for most factory workers, it lasts for 14 days. The duration is long because it is the only time of the year that people can go back, by all means available, to their own home to see their parents and be reunited with families, which can be the spouse and the children, since a significant portion of any urban population is made up of these people, called migrant workers. It is the only occasion when all families will try their best to get together to celebrate a family union. It is a deep rooted and endearing tradition. This is just like the UK, which has a population of slightly over 60 million, where everyone wishes to go home for Christmas or in the USA, with a population of 331 million, where everyone wishes to go home at Thanksgiving, to reunite with their families for a week or so. In China, this means 1.4 billion people.

Take this into context, then let us think about the situation in Wuhan. The infection was spreading, hospitals were completely overwhelmed and those who could afford it started to move out of Wuhan. The only way – and I can think of no other way, even with the wisdom of hindsight – to prevent the crisis from spreading was to lockdown the city completely. The city was locked down on January 23 and the first day of the Lunar New Year was January 25. This is a decision of the most daring and decisive kind. Only the Central Government in Beijing could make such an audacious decision. To me, it is a classic demonstration of the old cliche: damned if you do and damned if you don't. It was a Hobson's choice but a choice that had to be made, however uncomfortable and unprecedented it may be. The Western press was shocked by this lockdown. This has never happened before, where a modern urban city with 11 million people was shut down, let alone two days ahead of the most important day of the annual calendar. In simple terms, the public was told to stay at home and there was no alternative. All exits and entries to Wuhan were blocked and guarded. If someone was suspected with an infection, the patient would be admitted to a new hospital, built in 10 days, equipped with isolation wards. This was a complete and collective isolation of 11 million people with no one in and no one out, except for special personnel with PPE for the supplies of essentials. Chinese military took an active part in helping with the logistics. There was no problem with law and order but there was fear and desperation. The logistics of sustaining life fell on the shoulders of the military, police and above all, the brave front line medical and nursing staff in the hospitals. The Chinese government relocated a total of 50,000 medical doctors and nurses from all over the country to go there to help. Touchingly, nearly all went on a voluntary basis with only one intention in mind: to help their helpless compatriots in Wuhan.

I was also shocked at the time too by its audacity. But I also realized that this must be a very serious outbreak of epic historical significance for such a measure to be taken, just two days before the Lunar New Year. I was planning to go back to Shenzhen to the Hong Kong University Shenzhen Hospital where I work as a haematologist. Most colleagues, and my family, out of concern for my safety, advised me not to go back. But I did have my own professional concern as I am in charge of the bone marrow transplant programme in the hospital and knowing that as China entered the peak of the crisis from early February, there would be an acute shortage of blood and blood product supplies as people would simply stay at home. In other words, there would not be any blood donations. I had to manage the situation by suspending the marrow transplant programme until it was safe to restart. Delegating this responsibility to some other senior haematologist was of course an alternative for me but somehow I felt it would be more appropriate if I could explain to the patients myself as their lives were just as precious as those affected by Covid-19.

I arrived back at HKU SZH on February 4 and as well as being responsible for the haematology and bone marrow transplant programme, I soon became part of the medical team responsible for looking after all the suspected patients with Covid-19 in the isolation wards. For the six weeks I stayed in the hospital, I could not go to see my ageing mum of 96 in Hong Kong because Hong Kong closed the border with China and there was a mandatory 14 days quarantine. I saw and experienced at first-hand how China and in particular, Shenzhen and our own hospital, fought the virus. Without wanting to go into much detail, I was impressed, I was moved and I felt privileged to be there. There was no panic, no fear, but a single minded, unquestionable determination to get through this. Every time I thought about this experience, many faces and names cropped up in my mind.

By the time I left China on March 16, the airports in China and Hong Kong were virtually all in lockdown. I was fortunate that I was able to take a flight, through tortuous routes, back to the UK to rejoin my wife and son. By then, I was relieved to see that the outbreak was getting under control in China but then Italy became the epicentre.

When I got back to the UK, the outbreak was just about to enter its peak. The modelling showed that the infection and death toll would be higher than Italy. The UK went into lockdown a week after I came back, on March 23. Then the USA, mainly New York, became the epicentre. By the end of May, the UK and most European countries had passed the peak. The total global affected cases had reached the 6 million mark and recorded more than 360,000 deaths, with a mortality rate, based just on these two figures, of about 0.6%. The debates then were when and how to reopen the economy and how to balance that with the risk of emergence of the second wave if restrictions were lifted too early.

On reflection, with all the talk about tests and their debates, PPE and their shortages, herd immunity and its uncertainties, and the non-availability of specific drugs and vaccines, I would argue that in my view, lockdown was by far the single most effective measure used by most countries, painful though it is, in this crisis. This lockdown plus the public willingness to adhere to social isolation were the key factors for those of us who have sailed through by not catching the infection. Some had sadly lost their lives or their loved ones, but most of us are still alive. However high the economic cost may be, saving lives the way we did would at least give us a fighting chance to recover the economy too.

However, the story does not end there. Global crisis always has huge impact which can affect individuals, communities and nations. The nature of any outbreak, be it a fire or an earthquake or in this case, a virus, is that it can happen, again and again. But when it happens, it is often very unpredictable and sudden, however clever the forecasters may be. One can warn about all these crises but one cannot predict with confidence exactly when all these will happen. Such things are all acts of nature, and we should work together to deal with this as such.

And yet, in barely a few months since the start of the pandemic, even when the crisis was at its peak, there was the emergence of some extremely unhelpful, inaccurate and even mischievous views coming out from various corners. There were finger pointing, accusations and counter accusations, rumour mongering, almost like mud-slinging. These were the sort of behaviours unbecoming of leaders and politicians. Some of these were played out almost in real time in this age of social media, full of mischievous editing of sensational video clips and the spreading of fake news. They had one and only one purpose, that is, to seed hate, to lay blame on others and in so doing, incite animosity, and even racialism towards others in the most partisan way one can imagine. Just at the moment when countries needed to help and understand each other, they started to blame each other.

We all know that the virus started in Wuhan in China, then spread across China and then the rest of the world. One can say China may be the source, but it would be completely wrong and irresponsible to hint or even suggest that it was created by China. China was the loser here too, just like the rest of the world. Why would a country create something to destroy itself, just before the Lunar New Year? No one, despite the superb intelligence gathering capacity of the Five Eyes (the English-speaking countries of the USA, Canada, Australia, New Zealand and the UK), actually came out with any proof of any conspiracy or engineering of an accidental leak of virus from Wuhan. In this world of fake news, innuendo will suffice. Rumour will spread so quickly and become self-perpetrating, thanks to the social media. So however ridiculous these innuendoes may be, they will help to generate bigotry. There are people whose motives were to blame others to cover up for their own shortcomings. This was classically played out shamelessly and distastefully. Led by the USA, China-bashing, sadly, started to appear on the global political scene.

There were even suggestions that those affected countries should get together to sue China in the international court to seek compensation for the damage.

These were loose talks dismissed by the seriously minded. Sadly, such loose talks were put forward by the opportunists! In international laws, there is this clause called sovereign immunity, which means that one sovereign country cannot sue another sovereign country. Thankfully, the vast majority of serious statesmen, politicians, opinion shapers and academics treat such talks as noises to be ignored rather than to respond to. It was a non-starter, to be seen as a cynical attempt to shift the blame from an ill prepared administration to another country, so the public anger could be redirected at another country.

Another political debate was the suggestion that there should be an independent commission of enquiry into how and why the outbreak occurred in Wuhan. Again, this was another knee jerk reaction which cannot be taken seriously. First, how would the enquiry be funded? Then, what would be the terms of reference and how would these terms be decided? Who should carry out such an enquiry? So where will the independence be coming from? A selection of an international team of learned lawyers perhaps? Where would they be from and how would they be selected? Independent enquiry of course is very valuable in learning the lessons which need to be learned, but it works only within a sovereign country. Therefore, it is much more feasible and helpful to set up some sort of professionally and academically led international conference where people can share information with one another and to agree on consensus and future directions, rather than enquiry.

Perhaps one can put the argument the other way round. Twelve years ago, in the summer of 2008, we had the global financial crisis. It started in Wall Street. First there was the collapse of a bank called Bear Stearns which was then acquired by JP Morgan Chase at the request by the US Treasury. Then the crisis got out of hand, and Lehman Brothers collapsed in September 2008. Even for Lehman Brothers here was a desperate effort by the US Treasury to do another Bear Stearns but this time all the big investment bankers could not agree on a price and Lehman collapsed in September. It was only when, within a few days, the conglomerate of all conglomerates, the AIA, went through a similar trouble of being on the edge of collapse that it was felt by the US government that the banks were 'too big to fall' and if not handled properly, it would be spreading from Wall Street to High Street. So not only the financial sector would be destroyed, but the real economy too. The US government then stepped in to buy all the so-called toxic debts. They were called toxic for the simple reason that they will never be repaid. By then, in just six months, the world had got a full-blown financial crisis on its hands, even though some had warned of the crisis the year before, in 2007, because the root of the crisis, the subprime mortgages, was already in trouble as the US housing market started its slowdown.

It is widely accepted that the creation and the origin of the crisis was in the USA, starting with the subprime mortgages, where everyone with no credit would be hard sold a mortgage. In the years leading up to 2008, everyone wished to jump onto the mortgage bandwagon of owning a house. There was a housing boom with easy money. The mortgage lenders, out of their greed for commissions, helped to fuel the fire. The borrower's inability to pay back the loan would be ignored as the housing market would simply go up, and up and up, so their loan could be more than covered by the rise in their asset price, in that case, their house price. They were told by the mortgage lenders: don't worry, buy now and your house would be worth so much more than any mortgage interest you owe. Yes, money does not grow on trees but your money will grow from your house. It made the unsuspecting buyers feel dizzy that they were sitting on a pile of money, even though they hardly understood the way the loan was structured for them with the initial irresistibly short-term low interest rate. This was of course a twisted financial incentive. The mortgage providers, which were the banks, then passed their liability on the loans to the clever people in Wall Street. The clever people in Wall Street then spliced these loans up and created collections of assets of loans called bundles, known as credit swap derivatives, trading this as a kind of commodities or new kind of paper-based certificates, with a monetary value, between investment bankers, hedge fund managers and any greedy investors who wanted to join in this wonderful merry-go-round of inflating paper assets. Many got rich simply by hard selling these with trade-specific, fast-talking jargon to make them sound professional, in their usually suave and impressive tailor-made suits to make them look successful, to anyone who was just as greedy. None of these people would want to miss an opportunity like this of making fast money simply by making phone calls and pressing a few buttons on a keyboard for fast electronic trades. In this process of buying and selling on Wall Street, it should be noted that nothing tangible was actually created or manufactured, but just trading on a bundle of financial derivatives and jargon which no one, including the traders, really understood. So a bubble was created, and ended in the way bubbles always end. They burst into nothing. The trick was caught out finally as the lies could not be told any more. Anyone who was still in the bubble was exposed. By then the rich would have already made their millions, without having to do a single thing. Some greedy people were then left with assets which were truly toxic, as on paper these were valueless. Investment banks such as Lehman Brothers suddenly realized that not only had they nothing worthy to sell, but also no one could be fooled into buying it either. Furthermore, they didn't have any credit to borrow too. So this turned the gigantic credit crunch into the full-blown international financial crisis of 2008. In the end, some national governments, mainly the US and the UK, had to print money to get out of the crisis but the ordinary people, not the rich, had to suffer years of austerity. By the end of 2008, the world knew exactly where it occurred, who were involved and how it occurred. Yet 12 years later, as far as I know, not a single person or institution was successfully sued and found guilty of wrongdoings. One is not even sure if there was ever a public enquiry. One wonders why!

The events in 2008 were described in detail here for a reason. Just like Covid-19, it was seen as a global crisis. The reason for the crisis was unambiguous. In short, the crisis was initially generated by the banks and subsequently perpetuated by Wall Street. Yet very strangely, in a country where litigation is long regarded as the only way to correct rightness from wrongness, nothing came out of it except banks being bailed out, some directors being sacked. There was no independent enquiry. Even the British Monarch Queen Elizabeth II was rumoured to have raised in a meeting: why did no one see it coming? Well, in fact, a few did see it coming and had warned people as such, but their warnings were brushed aside. Her Majesty may feel entitled to ask of her subjects again: why did no one see this viral attack coming?

Covid-19 is not a crisis arisen out of greed, nor out of conspiracy. It was not a man-made financial crisis manufactured over a few years of relentless and aggressive lending. Covid-19 came out as an epidemic, an act of nature. It then became a global health crisis not seen since 1918, the year of the Spanish flu. It was a crisis which exploded onto the world scene in barely a few months. Did anyone see it coming? The answer is no, no one did. Did anyone then try to warn others after it happened? The answer is yes. Within four weeks, China notified the WHO in January 2020 and the WHO in turn warned the world. Did anyone take any serious notice after the WHO warning? All facts and figures suggested that no one did. There was complacency all round. This is precisely why, if there were to be any further studies of this crisis, they need to be open, impartial, dealing with facts and scientifically conducted with no preconceived assumptions. Above all, this must be free from political manipulation.

There is perhaps a certain degree of hypocrisy here. Instead of dealing with the crisis and looking after the public, some politicians attempted to divert their sole attention from fighting the virus to looking for the culprits beyond their own national boundaries, with the cynical intention of shifting the blame. Leadership starts at home and not by blaming others.

China was the first country to go through this pain and I have personally lived through the experience there. Then I lived through the same experience again in my adopted country, the UK, after I left China. It is fair to point out that as the UK was heading into the peak of the crisis, the government was honest enough to admit to the public that the NHS might be overwhelmed, the capacity to tests and thus contact tracing was severely limited, the supplies of PPE and ventilators were at dangerously low levels, not to mention the unachievable task of asking the people to wear masks (the public simply did not know where and how to get masks). With all these inadequacies, the British press roundly condemned the delayed and initial pathetic response from the government. They based their criticism by pointing out the time lapse from the global warning issued by the WHO on the events unfolding in Northern Italy in late February 2020, and then the speed at which the whole of Italy was in lockdown. The British press was asking the key question of what the government did or did not do from late January to early March. The same questions were also asked by the press in the USA of their government. This clearly demonstrated that nearly all countries had initial difficulties and delays in dealing with the virus. China had an initial delay too, from late December to mid-January.

Despite all the difficulties that the UK faced, while

suffering with the second highest death tolls in the West, after the USA, during Covid-19, the stoical acceptance and compliance of the British public with the government's advice was in my view the main reason that the peak was passed by the end of May. The UK government did have shortfalls in its response but the public realized the only realistic and practical measures that the government could take was total lockdown of the country, social distancing and self-isolation, as all the other measures that could be undertaken in other countries could not be undertaken for their logistical difficulties.

In short, what the UK government did and what many other countries did, though some would never admit it, was uncannily similar to what China did. When the crisis first broke out in Wuhan in December 2019, the Wuhan government and the Central Government were caught unprepared. Their absolute priority then was to confirm a possible outbreak first, then study the science, and then share the information globally with the WHO in accordance with its guidelines to its member states of reporting outbreaks of epidemics. At the same time, they had to decide on how to deal with this outbreak. The Chinese government also notified the US government before they informed the WHO officially. All these were done in the four weeks before the Spring Festival in late January 2020. There were uncertainties and confusion during the early phase of the outbreak. Information had to be carefully verified and vetted, or else the public would panic. The impartial observers, judging events over the subsequent six months with hindsight, could rightly conclude that there was no political ill intention from the Chinese government to deceive the world. Being the first country to suffer the crisis, China was caught off guard even more so than the other countries were subsequently. The people who would be the cheerleaders in pointing their fingers were often the same people who showed complacency and arrogance in February and early March in facing up to the pandemic, despite being forewarned by their own experts. Reassuring the public at the initial stage was of course necessary but it must be done with honesty, treating the public with respect and intelligence, and not with dismissive bravado. Reassuring the public by smearing the others, thus deceiving the public, was distasteful. Would the public see through this falsehood? No one knows. I hope they do. History will be the judge.

In this world, the East and the West co-exist. We learn from each other, we admire each other, we enrich each other, and we often help each other. In the case of Covid-19, perhaps one is allowed to opine that the West can learn from the East. Learning is never ever unidirectional; to think that one side has nothing to learn from the other side is truly the height of folly, arrogance and stupidity. In history, it is always the side which failed to learn that ended up being the loser.

CHAPTER 11

The Role of the WHO

The World Health Organization (WHO) is a specialized agency of the United Nations responsible for the international promotion of public health. It was established in 1948 and has 194 member states. The profile of the WHO has been raised significantly since Covid-19 when China first notified it, as a member state, of the outbreak of Coronavirus atypical pneumonia in Wuhan at the end of 2019. The WHO then sent a delegation to China to assess the outbreak and its Director General met with President Xi of China on January 28, 2020. Two days later, on January 30, 2020, the WHO issued a Public Health Emergency of International Concern (PHEIC). On February 11, the WHO named the outbreak officially as Covid-19. And on March 12, 2020, the WHO declared Covid-19 as a pandemic.

In the very early phase of the outbreak when it was mainly localized in China and some Asia countries, the WHO actively engaged with the Chinese authorities on the various ways of dealing with the outbreak. China saw the WHO as an impartial organization to share information with and seek advice from. However, since then the crisis became a pandemic with advanced economies bearing the brunt of the highest number of cases and death tolls. By late April, the USA became the country hardest hit by the pandemic in terms of numbers, with 1.2 million affected cases and more than 70,000 deaths. By the end of July 2020, the USA was reporting almost 4.5 million plus cases with almost 150,000 deaths. During this period, the USA was struggling with providing hospitals with enough PPE, ventilators and masks, which were all in short supply. Some states coped better than others, but the State of New York was particularly hit hard as it became the epicentre. Moreover, there was also confusion on what the responsibilities of the states are, and where the power of the states ends and where it starts with the federal government. In the USA, each state is responsible for many of its own affairs, especially healthcare. In dealing with the national crisis, where most of the populated states were caught unprepared, some senior government officials and politicians tried to shift the focus by looking for scapegoats and blamed China for the outbreak. Since China and the USA are the big two in this world and already at loggerheads with each other due to the tariff and trade disputes in the previous two years, China was a natural target for further US hostility. This happened at the worst possible time as China was coming out of the crisis and was opening up the country just when the USA was faced with the peak and being closed down. This was further inflamed when President Trump, after first complimenting the way China was handling the crisis in January 2020, changed his tune by targeting China a few times when the crisis in the USA was the epicentre in April 2020. Even his senior officials, especially his Secretary of State Mr Pompeo, made several disingenuous statements to that effect too. Not surprisingly, there were some public anti-China protests and even racial incidents in the USA. It must be stressed though that this anti-China tendency was not a mainstream phenomenon. There was nonetheless a tit-for-tat, and war of words between the two countries.

With that geopolitical background, the WHO unfortunately was caught in the crossfire. It made its assessment on China in January 2020, before the USA even realized it had a problem, and globally commended China for its efforts to deal with the outbreak. This may have clearly irked some of those in the West at precisely the moment the West was heading towards the peak of the crisis. A classic demonstration of the clique: if you

don't like the message, blame the messenger. The WHO
was making an assessment apolitically on China but
some countries complained that the WHO was too biased
and blind-sided by China. These were unfair criticisms
levelled against the WHO. The criticisms went further.
Every attempt by China to help other countries was
labelled as Diplomacy of Generosity by some. China, in
its eagerness to help, clearly was baffled by the signals
it received from other countries, mainly from the West.
The Chinese people did not understand quite how their
gestures of help were misconceived as cynical and publicity
seeking. These two different views, one from China and
the other predominantly from the West, led to further
misunderstanding. It was one of the most disappointing
and unnerving issues in this whole pandemic. Meanwhile,
the WHO was busy issuing warnings to the world but
also came under some unfair criticisms too. Had the
relationship between the G2 countries been better, the
political fallout would be much more manageable. As
it was, it put the WHO under some unfair criticism and
pressure amidst what has been described as a 'diplomatic
balancing act' between 'China and China's critics'. These
allegations even included the demands for a closer scrutiny
of the relationship between the WHO and the Chinese
authorities. These allegations were clearly wide of the
mark. The situation was further inflamed by threats that

the funding to the WHO would be withdrawn, just when
the WHO was busy helping and advising its member states
in the fight against Covid-19. The West's main concern
was over the reliability and the speediness of the data
provided by the Chinese authorities to the WHO. Again,
this allegation was unproven. Each country does have its
own way of collecting and validating data. For example, in
the UK, there were widespread criticisms from the national
press about the death tolls in the country, which was higher
compared with other countries in the West. The UK public
was told repeatedly by government officials that every
country has its own ways of collecting and analysing data.
Even in the USA, there was emergence in May of rumours
of displeasure from the White House with the way the data
was collected and analysed by each state. To criticize the
same thing about China and the WHO seems unfair. Data
itself does not lie, it was just a figure; what may differ is
how one collects and interprets the data. So the WHO, an
apolitical internationally recognized organization, in trying
to put in its best efforts in the face of a global pandemic,
now found itself in a situation where the number one
funding source, the USA, was threatening to withdraw
its funding by the president pending further assessments
of the WHO to be carried out by the USA. In expressing
its displeasure, the USA used the word 'China-centric' to
criticize the WHO. In other words, the funding will only

be secured if the WHO becomes more centric towards its biggest paymaster. The WHO, based in Geneva, is already full of experts from various institutions in the USA, such as the National Institute of Health and the Center for Disease Control and Prevention. So there is no lack of US representation there to suggest that the WHO is too China-centric with the implied message that the USA was not adequately represented in the WHO. It is also worth pointing out that, not too widely known to the public, the second biggest source of funding to the WHO is the Bill and Melinda Gates Foundation, a charitable US institution. Mr Bill Gates has recently stated openly that the WHO needs to be supported.

This geopolitical tension has ensnared the WHO into a distraction not through its own making. The Director General himself does not have the power to overturn the decision of the member states. The current Director General is a soft spoken, mild mannered Ethiopian. He was elected by the member states to run a technical and scientific organization. He has to grease the hinge of the door connecting the rich and the poor, and in so doing, the poor can have a voice. He also has the job of keeping international efforts alive when vaccine nationalism is already being openly discussed. Furthermore, he has himself faced constant, often personal and ugly, racial harassments online.

Advocates of the WHO have suggested by staying out of politics, it may allow the WHO to have an opportunity to persuade some secretive and repressive regimes in Africa to open the door so that its scientists, experts and doctors can work together across borders and save lives. Currently, only the WHO can carry out such a role. After all, it does have 72 years of experience since its inception in 1948.

All institutions will of course need reforms regularly to improve but such reforms do not for a minute negate the necessity of the WHO. In fact, the Director General agreed that the WHO needs to undertake a review on how improvements can be made. This is proper governance required in any organization and the need is self-evident without the interference from politics. Just imagine a situation if the WHO is disbanded or becomes defunct from 2021 onwards and then one year later the pandemic happens again, or if another Ebola outbreak happens in a poor country in Africa, who would raise the alarm and coordinate all the work across countries to help a country in a health crisis? The key point here is: either each country pursues its own policy or the world sets up a globalized institution to play a key role. In the case of Covid-19, the USA seems quite confident that it can do it all alone by having the right treatments, the right vaccines and the right tests, all marketed by US companies with priorities given to the US citizens. A more realistic and plausible scenario is that all countries can collaborate with one another, especially the rich ones such as China, Germany, France, Japan, South Korea, Italy and the UK, in coming up with the right treatments, right vaccines and right tests, backed up by an efficient logistics of supply chains not only to help their own people but also those in the poor countries too. If the world does wish to pursue such a sensible policy in a collaborated way in the world stage, especially in a pandemic like Covid-19, where or what is the institution of sufficient experience and legitimate representation of the poor countries which can take on such a role, if not the WHO? The race for treatment and vaccine is a race between the rich countries to claim the top prize because of the prestige and fortunes it will bring, but then other than that, wouldn't the poor countries deserve our help too? There needs to be a voice for the poor countries, especially on health matters, and the WHO can provide that voice.

In a major gesture of support for the WHO, President Xi of China announced, via a live video broadcast at the opening session of the WHO Annual Assembly on May 18, 2020, that China would support an investigation into the handling of the Covid-19 pandemic, and that any inquiry should not be commenced until the virus is contained globally. He also suggested that this investigation should be scientifically and professionally led, and the scope of the investigation must be comprehensive, involving international participation, led and coordinated by the WHO. Furthermore, he backed up China's support for the WHO by pledging that China would allocate US$2 billion over two years to help affected countries, particularly developing countries, in their Covid-19 response. On the very same day, Mr Azar II, the US Secretary of Health and Human Resources, also via a prerecorded video broadcast to the same Assembly of the WHO, sharply criticized the WHO by saying that its handling of the outbreak in China had led to unnecessary deaths. This was a serious and hitherto unfounded allegation against an organization which is professionally led with a charter granted to it by the United Nations.

During this crisis, few governments in the world, certainly outside of Asia, can claim to have handled the pandemic in an exemplified way. Almost all had been caught unprepared and inevitably mistakes had been made. However, all governments, without exception, did try to do their best on such a seismic event which most had not had previous experience in. The public understood and accepted this. In the UK, it had been widely viewed by the public and the press that the care home excess death was a national scandal, and the UK government had admitted to the problem and started to deal with it in earnest. What was unacceptable was to pass the blame onto another institution without accepting that governments themselves were less than perfect in handling the crisis. At best, it can be seen as shifting the blame. At worst, it could be seen as a cynical and systematic attempt to turn the issue into a political game for political gain. In dealing with Covid-19, nearly all countries have made mistakes, perhaps less so for a few in Asia, but it does not help to solve any problem if one country is singled out for blame.

The WHO is a globalized institution, and yet it has been caught against the headwind in the present climate of finding fault lines in globalization. Fundamentally, I believe that the WHO is a force for good and the ideals enshrined in the WHO are noble, idealistic and altruistic. It can help to bring the health level of the people in this world to a higher level while it can also act as a leveller for health inequalities. Like any institutions with good governance, it is self-evident that there will always be room for improvement. But it does not mean one needs to break everything it does for the sake of one member state's political or geopolitical preference.

All the important global institutions, such as the UN, the WHO, the World Bank, and the IMF need the support of the USA as it is the undisputed leader of the world. These organizations will be much the poorer without the support, participation and leadership provided by the USA. There should always be a family head in any families and the USA is the head of the families of nations. The USA's agenda of 'America First' should be considered in the right context. The USA is already first in so many areas and on so many fronts. One only needs to take a look around the inside of any university, a hospital, a well provided home, a bank, a mobile device, or take a trip to cyberspace, then pause to have a think. One will soon realize how far ahead of everyone else and dominant the USA is. To many around the world, the USA is a country most would look up to admiringly. Its openness, its popular and imaginative Hollywood blockbusters, its science and technology achievements, its innovation and its medical advances, are all leading the pack. Never mind its hard power, its soft power is second to none and possibly unrivalled in human history. It makes the rest of us marvel at the talents of that young, dynamic and multicultural country. It is a matter of envy and admiration from the rest of the world that the USA has the most Nobel Laureates in all its categories. It consistently occupies the top spot over the years. In 2019, it has 383 Nobel Laureates, more than the combined total of the next 4 countries on the top five list! So many of us want to learn from it, and even be like it. The influence it has with its soft power can be felt and seen in all corners of the world. The talents and the collective might that the USA generates are the real intangible gains of the unrivalled soft power the country enjoys on a global scale. Every time the world went through a crisis, be it a war, a financial meltdown, an embargo by the oil cartels, the war on terrorism, the USA has always come out stronger, and never weaker. I have not personally come across any informative study demonstrating that the USA is weaker as a result of the challenges it has faced over the years. Quite the contrary, the USA has always demonstrated its remarkable ability to keep reinventing itself. This undisputed strength of the USA should not be and cannot simply be equated with or measured by a set of figures of trade deficit with one country or its financial contribution to international institutions. The real gains are often unquantifiable. In addition, power needs to be earned and exercised wisely. It also comes with obligation and discipline. That power is most awesome and sustainable if it is admired and not resented by others. In other words, the USA would be well advised not to be aiming to be, or burdened with, being first in absolutely everything and anything. It puts others under constant pressure to catch up in this interconnected world and above all, it puts itself under unnecessary and imaginary pressure. Let others prosper a bit and the USA can prosper more. Does it really matter to the winning team if the soccer match is won by 6-1 instead of 6-0? I believe it does not, but it will offer the opponents a bit of consolation by scoring a single and consolation goal.

It is therefore a matter of huge regret that the USA is now adopting such a negative attitude towards the WHO.

Whatever the criticisms and reservations about the WHO, this is quite possibly the worst time to negate its effort and contribution. By late July 2020, the affected cases in the world have breached 15 million and the WHO pleaded for global solidarity and leadership. The WHO itself does not have the mandate to lead. We do now need leader(s) and still to this day the global community would hope that the USA would continue to lead. No time is more important than the present time to steer the world away from indecision and division, as failure to reach global consensus will only lead to more infection and more deaths.

CHAPTER 12

The New Normal

It is now generally predicted and accepted that the world the day after Covid-19 will be different from the day before. Due to the extent of the pandemic, and the scale of the changes that each country has to make in order to deal with this crisis and to prepare for the future crisis, at least some changes will be permanent. These new changes are now known as the New Normal. In some countries such as China, South Korea and Italy, which had opted to start reopening their countries from early May 2020, it was already clear that there were some significant permanent changes both institutionally and socially.

Let us start with shopping first. Retail industries and shopping malls were running into some major difficulties even before Covid-19. Some major household names were scaling down. The main reason for this was always thought to be the expansion in both the scope and scale of online shopping, which offers the sort of convenience that no shopping malls can match. Big fashions shops such as Marks & Spencer and Top Shop in the UK were already closing stores, as a result of the huge growth and intense competition from online shops. The new trend of social behaviour emerging after Covid-19 may put a further strain on them. It has already been proven in China at the height of the crisis that people could shop adequately without going to the shops. Since the gradual re-opening of China to business, it was apparent that shopping malls continued to struggle even for those who were thriving before the crisis. There are two main reasons for this change. The first reason is that the Chinese have always embraced online shopping with excellent O2O (online to offline) service. The logistics support for such O2O service has been the most efficient system that I have personally experienced. This includes track and delivery, and products return. During the height of the crisis in China, I remember once I had to order online from my mobile app some food and toiletries, with free delivery if the total was over RMB 30 (about GBP 3), and I was able to get my stuff in 35 minutes. So one does not really need to go to the mall to shop as all the stuff the mall can offer will be available online, perhaps with more choices too. Before Covid-19, shopping malls were crowded as most people, especially the young, would see the experience not only as shopping but rather an occasion for dining and socializing with friends. That is, going to the malls was a social experience to be enjoyed as a leisure activity. This can be lumped as social and consumer activities merging into one, especially during weekends. The leisure and retail industries have always been an important sector for economic growth as the Chinese government started to encourage consumer spending over the last few years. After the shock of Covid-19, however, when buzzing cities like Shanghai, Beijing and Shenzhen started to open, it is obvious that while some visitors are coming back, they are spending less. Restaurants, especially the expensive ones at the top end of the market, seem to have fewer customers. Surveys carried out to assess this New Normal found that most people, even after recovery from Covid-19, were planning to cut down on shopping and spending, even for the affluent young urban dwellers with high earnings. They felt more insecure about the economic outlook and wished to save more. In addition, they also recognized the hazards of crowds and so there is now a new culture of avoiding being too close to each other even when socializing. So the idea of social distancing has truly set in as a trend, not as a measure to combat Covid-19 but as a sign of good personal habit to prevent any droplet infections.

In addition to this, wearing masks will be much more common. I dare to predict that masks will be colourful and personalized too. I think countries like China, South Korea, Japan and Singapore in the East and France in the West will be trendsetters. I think this new trend will catch on very quickly globally and soon it will be a social norm for wearing masks, even in the West. There is now an almost universal agreement that masks will offer some protection from infection. After Covid-19, these trends of fewer people in shopping malls and more people wearing masks will be the new normal. What about eating out, which all of us enjoy? It is likely that the restaurants are changing their business model too. They would not allow diners all squeezing in around a small table. Bookings for a table for four may now have a new meaning. There could be real difficulties here as the restaurant owners have to make more space for fewer people. Spreading people apart more can only mean less business and higher costs. On the other hand, some restaurants clearly may take matters of public health as a priority to protect both the customers and the staff. In China, the public has already been asked to have an app on their mobile phone in which one can check on a QR code which will indicate in colour and in real time the health status of a person. A green colour would indicate permission for freedom of movements (green to go), and red colour indicating high risk and movements are to be severely restricted (red to stop). As a result, some restaurants in China are already requiring the customers to show on the mobile phone their health status. Only those showing a green colour on the app are allowed to go in. So it is like a passport or traffic lights for dining in public. Indeed, they may well be extended to shopping malls, leisure parks or cinemas. Even in the posh restaurants, gone will be the days when all the cutlery or chopsticks would be nicely set and displayed on the table, but rather they would come when the dishes are being served. It is quite possible the menu will be reduced too to avoid the risk of cross infections between too many ingredients contaminating each other.

Other changes in the service industries are that if we do go to the restaurants or bars or shops, it is likely that those who serve us will be wearing gloves and masks. In fact, those who do this are likely to have more customers. If someone invites me out for dinner, then I would prefer to go to a restaurant where the staff there wear masks, gloves or even aprons, as part of a welcoming and colour coordinated uniform, to make the ambience feel less like a hospital canteen. The bar tenders, who were so used to chatting with the customers, may from now on have their face half covered for their own protection. I can even see that when people go to watch a new blockbuster film, no one will go in without masks. In short, those manufacturers who make masks will have a growing business, it will no longer be surgical masks that will be in demand, but protective masks made like a new fashion accessory will be in demand more. Masks should therefore help to make leisure activities more fun and less inconvenient. In airport terminals, at check-in counters, the passengers would almost certainly be required to wear masks and in fact the customs and border control officers would wear masks too! It is only when one goes through the security gate or passport control that one would be asked to take the mask off. When I returned to the UK in March, I had to be reminded by the passport control to remove my mask – that was because it was before the lockdown, so anyone wearing a mask going through border checkpoint was seen as strange, or even suspicious! I am sure it would be strange no more next time when I pass through, it would indeed be strange if no one wears a mask. The flight attendants will certainly wear masks and I will feel safer if they do since they will serve us with food and beverages. This conversion of wearing masks after Covid-19 somehow as the norm is one of the unexpected consequences leading to the Easternization of the West. The Westernization of the East in the last 200 years does seem to have a reverse gear after all. It is interesting to note at least two famous columnists, one in the USA, and one in the UK, both writing in well-respected international newspapers, admitted in their own columns that they were sent masks and PPE from their friends in Beijing, and both columnists appreciated this and found having these masks quite reassuring. Some of my friends in Hong Kong also sent masks by express delivery to their families in the USA. I myself was also sent masks by friends in China and Hong Kong. A levelheaded person will say that it does not really matter if the culture is east or west, as long as it helps to reduce the infection and improve public health, then that is what matters. There are other predictable changes for the new normal. We would not be provided with a fitting room when we go and select new clothes in a fashion shop. And if we go into a shoe shop, we certainly would not be allowed to try the shoes on. Gone are the days, especially in the top brand fashion shops, when one could try one outfit after another. And, when we do go to the supermarket for groceries, it is almost certain that we will need to queue at least one metre (it used to be two metres at the height of the crisis in the UK) apart from each other and wait for our turn to be allowed to go in. Couples shopping together or group shopping may not be allowed, unless it is someone with a creche carrying a small child. The space, even in a spacious supermarket, will not be allowed to get crowded; any chance for the spread of viral infection must be minimized.

So, the new shopping and leisure experience will be part of the new normal, because public health concerns will override public convenience. I cannot see how this will not be accepted willingly by the public. In fact, supermarkets going back to the old way may even be criticized by the public. On that note, I keep thinking about the situation in Hong Kong where the supermarkets are generally just one third of the size of their UK counterparts due to the scarcity of physical space with perhaps quadruple the number of customers who are often unavoidably bumping into each other. I wonder how the new normal can be accommodated there. Still, the people of Hong Kong have always been smart and ingenious, they will find a way.

All these changes are behavioural in nature, out of the need to protect oneself and those around us but one other thing I predict with confidence, which may also be the New Normal, will be a rapid move towards a cash-free society. In this respect, my experience leads me to think China is way ahead of most. I still carry my wallet with me and my mobile phone when I go out in China. But even though my mobile phone is a smartphone, I do not have an account in China to enable WeChat pay or Alipay, so I have to use either cash or credit card. The problems I had encountered for quite a few times is that in China, small businesses, such as taxi services doing small transactions, often do not take cash and certainly would not take credit cards, they would only take payment through WeChat pay or Alipay from the customer's mobile phone. This movement towards a cash-free society means that cash will be phased out. Paper and coins are totally unhygienic. One does not need a vivid imagination to guess just how many pairs of hands this cash has passed through before it lands onto your hand! Imagine also that just when you are taking cash out from your wallet and suddenly you sneeze, that would be really embarrassing. I would guess the other side may refuse to take my cash, and quite rightly too. Nothing untoward will happen to you of course but then think of the impact if you run a shop and that happens to you or one of the customers on a regular basis. Your shop may soon turn into a health hazard. This is why many shops in China do not take cash. Already in the UK, figures coming out from the UK had shown that the use of ATMs (automated teller machines) had gone down by 40%, and these days, I have hardly ever seen anyone in the supermarkets pay their grocery bills with cash.

All the above discussions have been on changes mainly to personal behaviour, but what about the new normal in mass gatherings such as sporting events, indoor or outdoor concerts, church activities? At the time of the writing of this book, it was not clear how this would be phased back into society. I would guess because it involves so many people all attending a scheduled, not spontaneous, event at the same time, then there will be an additional check and registration procedure, in addition to entry tickets, preferably using a tracking app on the mobile phones to clarify the health status of the attendees, much like the way they are doing in China. There may also be a need for mandatory temperature monitoring or wearing of facial coverings, and also certainly some rules of physical distancing from each other. If I jump up in joy when the Liverpool football team scores on the 89th minute and I go crazy (I am normally very cool) and bear hug the guy next to me, say who is sitting one metre away, I think I will either be punched by him, or even her, and the stewards in the stadium will ask me to leave and the club will impose the ultimate fine on me by banning me to future matches! For those music performers in a concert, one can safely assume the audience will likely be wearing masks. I can't imagine how though, if the Royal London Philharmonic Orchestra is playing Beethoven 9th in the Royal Albert Hall, the musicians could be wearing masks, or would they not? Would the masks get in the way of the violinists? And in a place of worship like churches, how would the Holy Communion be taken? In Japan, the government actually has issued guidelines on their popular activities. Those going to karaoke have to be kept two metres apart from each other and wear masks or shields except when they are drinking or singing. Those who go to game parlours, another popular pastime among the Japanese, have to keep the sound of the consoles at the lowest volume so that people do not have to shout over it. In fact, in the new normal, we will all have to talk quietly or even be prepared to repeat what we say because of the masks and the possible presence of a shield in between us and the other side.

The mode of international travel will be changed too, be it air, sea or land travel. For air travel, the new normal will almost certainly mean that flights will be less frequent, prices will go up and for some exotic destinations, it may not even be possible or become very cumbersome. Tourism will have a new meaning. A visitor booking into a 5-star hotel may check to ensure that the hotel practises a very stringent infection control process. I would also guess that it would take a long time for the international flights to get back to anywhere near where they were before Covid-19, if ever that is possible. The airline industry players themselves have predicted it will be at least 2025 before they can go back to the previous level of service. In designing new planes, would it be commercially viable to have seats apart? Some airlines are already thinking of abolishing the seats in the middle of the aisle. If so, the lost revenue can only be covered by significantly increasing the price of tickets. One area which is distinctly under threat is the luxury cruise travels. Even before the crisis, these cruises are expensive and tend to serve mainly the elderly and the affluent. In a modern day luxurious ocean liner, access to medical help is very limited. Could this mean that the modern luxurious cruise will need to be reconverted to have an ICU type of facilities just in case there is a potential outbreak? And if so, would this ICU be managed by qualified staff? All cruise travels will have the same problems to resolve as their journeys tend to be the longest, measured in days and not hours.

Another observation in the new normal is the way medical services, especially hospital services, will be run after Covid-19. It is already very clear that the public attitude to hospitals is changing. When I was in China in early February 2020, we noticed a sharp drop in outpatient attendances, partly because some services were closed, and there was also a sharp drop in inpatient services too. The primary aim of all these closures reflected a determination by the hospital management to reduce cross infection. Equally, the public may also feel that it may be safer to stay at home rather than attending a hospital which may increase their risk of infection. By mid-April in China, nearly all hospital services had returned to full capacity with no shortage of beds, no shortage of PPE and no shortage of tests, but the clinical activity was still significantly lower than before the crisis. The same phenomenon happened in Europe and the UK too. The great initial fear was that the UK health service, known as the NHS, would simply be overrun and doctors and nurses would get infected and go on sick leave. With fewer beds and staff to come in to deal with the clinical demands, the UK government slogan initially was: Stay home, save the NHS, save lives, meaning only staying home can save the NHS to save lives. It was scary then, not dissimilar to what happened in Wuhan in January 2020. Major cities like London were affected even worse. Other cities like New York in the USA also faced the same problems. The UK then came through April by the skin of its teeth. In May, the crisis passed its peak and it was then noticed that spare capacity in the non Covid-19 wards was not fully used up. Where the average bed occupancy rate in any major hospital used to be around 85% to 90%, it had dropped by a third to about 60%. Emergency Room (ER) attendances, which had always been a source of horror stories of patients in temporary beds waiting in the hospital corridors, were down by 50%! This has prompted calls for patients not to delay seeking attention in the ER where necessary; heart attacks and strokes were two classic areas of concern, as these are life threatening. This was something which was unheard of previously in my 30 years of serving the NHS. Before Covid-19, the public was often told hospitals could not cope because of overwhelming clinical demands, with the consistent message that hospital services were overused, especially in the ER. Now the pendulum has swung to the other extreme. The public now has a new view that home isolation may be safer than hospitals. As a result of this

underuse of non Covid-19 hospital services, the government
officials started to tell the patients in the media that they
must not avoid the hospital. The truth, in my view, is that
through the lessons of Covid-19, most of the public have
accepted that hospitals are mainly there for emergencies
and specialized care, and perhaps not the 'be all and end
all' of medical services as previously thought. The public
may now have also realized that chronic conditions such
as hypertension and diabetes really do not need hospital
care. A good primary care centre would be as good as any
in providing adequate service for these conditions. Another
plausible and altruistic reason is that they genuinely may
feel that by not going to the hospitals, they could help to
free up the staff to work in the more needed areas such as
ICU.

The same phenomenon has been reported in the USA
too. A poll released in the middle of May 2020 revealed
that the emptiness of medical care centres may also reflect
the choices patients made to delay care. The Kaiser Family
Foundation poll found that 48% of Americans said they
or a family member had skipped or delayed medical care
because of the pandemic, and 11% of them said the person's
condition worsened as a result of the delayed care. It did not
indicate in what way their medical conditions deteriorated
or in what disease groups they were referring to, though
nearly seven in 10 of those who had skipped seeing a

medical professional expected to get care in the next three months. Yet, despite a significant number of adults saying they delayed care, 86% of adults said their physical health has 'stayed about the same' since the onset of the outbreak in the USA. This is quite possibly the first and largest poll (involving more than 1,000 respondents) in trying to assess the phenomenon of non-attendance in hospitals or health centres. So this trend of using fewer healthcare services which I witnessed myself in China, the UK and the USA, has been broadly similar. This has caused a problem in a market-driven, demand-driven and technology-driven healthcare system like that of the USA, as it has resulted in grievous financial losses for hospitals and clinics. Medical practices have closed. Hospitals have been forced to furlough employees or cut pay.

However, there is yet a more troubling explanation to consider: Perhaps the public may not require the volume of care that their doctors are used to providing.

It is well recognized that a substantial amount of healthcare in the USA, and perhaps in the UK too, is wasteful and not clinically necessary but for the concerns of the patients that a diagnosis is not immediately apparent or the doctors practising defensive medicine to avoid litigations. This is perhaps more noticeable in the use of expensive diagnostic tests or treatments. There may be a lack of consensus and the belief that the newest and

the most expensive are always better. The overprovision
of the trendy tests or treatments may invariably involve
an unnecessary waste or inappropriate use of resources.
Free market in medicine may not be the best idea of
allocation of resources. The waste may account for not an
insignificant amount of the total healthcare budget. The
classic example one can use is the approach to back pain,
known as lumbago, which is very common and by far the
most common cause is due to musculoskeletal strain, and
yet often an MR scan is requested for such cases as one of
the first lines of investigations. Another example is the use
of expensive and extensive genetic tests to screen for the
possibility, not the presence, of cancers for someone who
does not have a strong family history of cancer. So Covid-19
may conceivably reveal that there may indeed be a wasteful
side of healthcare in its overprovision. This is a serious area
for the policymakers to take note of since the healthcare
budget is always the number one policy headache faced by
many countries as an area with an open and inexhaustible
demand, so any area which can reduce waste should be
welcome and considered.

On the provision of medical services and avoidance of
waste, one of the new normals will be the coming of age
of telemedicine, which was already discussed in Chapter
8. I am professionally quite used to it already because it
is fairly well practised in China and many hospitals are

offering teleconsultation. Other countries have now also realized that today not only the technology is fully mature and robust, it is also one of the safest ways to reduce cross infection. In the UK, the GPs are moving more and more towards telemedicine and the scope for this is tremendous. For instance, one can imagine a scenario where a 24/7 GP service can be available online, with the GP taking rota to staff it from home. Patients do not have to rely on their own transport or public transport to attend. There is another eco-friendly spin-off, which is, the record of the teleconsultation can be digitalized and stored via cloud technology as a documented evidence for any audit purposes. Most medical conditions actually do not require the traditional physical examination of the patient but may rather require further tests, which the GP can request via a secure app or secured website. I now ask for my own repeat prescriptions via my GP access app, and it is most efficient. This can also ensure that the consultation will be carried out in a safe, quiet and private environment. I am fairly convinced it will be welcome by all. We may have been too slow and reticent in taking this up, and before Covid-19 we would have not realized the full potential that telemedicine could offer. But the recent scare of the pandemic has given us a real opportunity to rethink the roles that telemedicine can play in personalized healthcare. There is now already an active debate in China on the feasibility of downloading personal medical information onto personal mobile devices. We must be prepared to see this as the new normal as an alternative plank of medical care, especially these days when test results and images can all be digitalized and viewed via secure links. Consultation should not be viewed as a must-be on site exclusive service in the health centre or hospital. A more secure, timely and auditable mobile device serves a much better and flexible purpose, and the aim here is not to replace the traditional consultation but to augment the efficiency and convenience of the service. So, gone will be the days when one could only see a doctor by appointment, which was somehow never ever at the time one wanted, or one could attend the ER, so there were only two choices on the menu. But the new normal at least can ensure there are more items on the menu for the patients to choose from.

I also noted that in April 2020, the world stock markets took a nosedive with some stocks such as the airlines and hotels industry dropping more than 50%. In fact, since the stock market investors like to think of themselves as smart people who know things before anyone, these drastic falls spooked governments all over the world into pumping an almost unlimited amount of money into the economy, using the words: whatever it takes to calm the markets and the public. Stock markets, not only being smart, efficient and quick, also deal with fear and greed. In this apocalyptic period of Covid-19, the virus has successfully instilled fear, over six months, into the public, the stock markets and the governments, all over the world, without exception. It was also reported in the press that the stock prices of the big techno giants, including the king of retailing and logistics, Amazon, not only did not fall, but had actually gone up. This was of course because the markets now realized how these techno giants had demonstrated that in a global crisis, what a dominating and indispensable role they can play for the public, the governments and their shareholders. The track and trace app in the UK was developed jointly by Google and Apple. They are the engines of further economic growth in the world. These apps are clean and infection-free. Ironically, the equivalence of hacking attacks on these giants and their apps are also called viral attacks. The words 'gone viral' are commonly used to describe that a piece of gossip or information has gone into the cyberspace with speed, and goes unchecked once someone puts it in the cyberspace, a bit like a true infective viral attack on the humans. However, I believe that the technical sophistication and vigilance of protecting themselves from cyberattacks, undertaken by these giants, will mean that any hacking will be noticed by these techno giants far quicker than any real viral attacks on humans, and dealt with much more quickly and effectively too. They can simply take it away from cyberspace by pressing a few

buttons. These giants can connect us all, and we must let
them play a key part in the protection of our collective
health too. I emphasized collective health in the sense that
it can serve as a regular and powerful tool to alert us in real
time when and where the new clusters are in any future
outbreaks, so we can stay away. In China, this is already
part of the new normal of using technology to protect us.
To put it more simply, we can each have a personal radar in
our own personal devices to check the environments for us,
we just need to be careful on the ethical and privacy side
of this to strike off an acceptable balance between public
health safety and our privacy.

Another serious area for discussion is what form
can education in future take? Internet-based teaching is
already part of the basis of primary, secondary and tertiary
learning. One of the advantages for this form of teaching
is that physical class size may not be a constraint, while
interactive teaching between teacher and students can
still be maintained. The popularity of a lecture will not
be judged by the size of the lecture hall where everyone is
sitting close to and next to each other. The teaching and
lecturing can be done far more safely and flexibly via the
internet. The University of Cambridge announced in May
2020 that all face-to-face lectures will cease for the whole
2020/2021 academic year. Invitation for luminaries from
overseas to give lectures in seminars and conferences can

be cheaper since they will not need to be provided with flights and hotels. The speakers will not suffer jet lag either. I am not suggesting conferences are not needed but the format for the conferences can be much more flexible and in line with the new normal. A professor may not wish to fly to an area where there may be an epidemic, but he may not decline a lecture delivered at his own home turf so that far more people can benefit from his knowledge. I already know some professors who have been giving more internet-based lectures than face-to-face lectures for many years.

CHAPTER 13

Why are Mortalities Higher in Richer Countries?

Nearly all countries with the highest number of affected cases belong to the G10 countries (not to be confused with G7, 8 or 20). G10 actually consists of 11 industrialized countries which share similar economic policies and which meet annually. They can be regarded as the closest 11 economic cousins in the world. To be precise, these are Belgium, Canada, France, Germany, Italy, Japan, the Netherlands, Sweden, Switzerland, the UK and the USA. Except Japan, all the countries are European or North American countries. In short, all rich countries; Japan of course is the only one included from the East.

The puzzling and yet challenging question is, despite

their vast individual and collective wealth for all these 11 sovereign countries, why was their death toll higher on a per capita basis, compared with some Asian countries such as China, Japan and South Korea? By the end of July 2020, China had a death toll of 4,634, Japan had a death toll of 1,913 and South Korea had a death toll of 301. By comparison, the USA had about 150,000 deaths, the UK had about 46,000 deaths, and Italy had a death toll of 35,000. The USA and the UK have the highest numbers of infective cases and deaths in the G10, closely followed by Italy, France and Spain. More worryingly, England's Office for National Statistics (ONS) announced on May 7 that in England, black people were four times more likely to die from Covid-19. Social scientists postulated that in these countries, black people generally tend to belong to the lower social economic class who often live in poor environments with substandard hygiene provisions. They are also in general employed in low paid jobs working in unsavoury environments, unable to protect themselves adequately as they may not have the means to. This is a real social problem which each government has to address. In stark contrast, if one looks at Asia in the same period, one is then struck by the much lower number of deaths in China, Vietnam and South Korea. On June 2, 2020, the PHE (Public Health England) confirmed that the BAME group also has higher mortalities. BAME refers to Blacks, Asians, and minority ethnicities. The PHE thus confirmed that for Covid-19, the risk groups are the elderly, male, those living in cities and BAME. The PHE also admitted this was only a statistical observation and made no attempt to assess why this was so, though the key stand out difference of the BAME is that they tend to be in the lower social economic class – in other words, poverty has something to do with it.

Apart from the social and economic reasons, I do think that to address the observation further, there ought to be a science-based study to find out the reasons why mortality affecting the black people and the BAME community as a whole is higher in the Covid-19 pandemic, despite them being citizens of the richest countries in the world. It is commonly thought the vast difference in infections, say between Japan or China (which is not in G10) in the East and the USA and UK in the West, is due to the early and comprehensive use of diagnostic tests, contact tracing, masks and other personal protections in the East, while those in the West did not prepare themselves properly by not paying sufficient early attention to the importance of such measures. But these measures may explain the difference in the total number of affected cases but not death toll, especially when the G10 countries are regarded as having the world's leading healthcare services in terms of skills, bed capacity and equipment, compared to countries like perhaps India and Vietnam. So it can be plausible that the BAME suffer more deaths not only because they are poor, but they did not have equal access to standard medical care because of the citizenship status. For instance, in the UK, one now has to prove resident status before one is entitled to free medical services. This possible access restriction to medical care faced by the BAME must be checked out by the PHE, which would have more thorough data on each of these patients who died.

A separate report from the ONS in England which suggested that black people are four times more likely to die also warrants special mention. If similar findings can be confirmed in other countries with a diverse cultural and ethnic mix such as the USA, and in cities like New York, where there is a significant black population, then it will be a very serious social economic problem which must be addressed. Soon after the early information from the ONS in England was released, similar information started to come out from New York City too, that black people also suffered from a higher death toll. This was then subsequently reported in other cities in the USA as well. There could be a genetic reason for it but genetic reason can only explain why the disease may be more common in the black population, not why it is more lethal, especially in countries with the world's best health system. For instance, sickle cell disease (a lifelong inherited blood condition in which the red cells are born with the wrong shape as a result of one amino acid mutation in the gene coding of the haemoglobin molecule, thus making the red cell more fragile and rigid) is more common in black people, but those sickle cell patients in the USA fare much better and live longer than those with the same disease in the Caribbean Islands or Africa. These patients in the USA and Canada have the highest standards of medical care compared with those from other countries. Their scientific research on this disease is second to none too. In other words, the USA is much better at looking after patients with sickle cell disease, a condition commonly found in black people. To truly find out why black people are suffering a higher death rate in Covid-19, much more effort must be made. If indeed the reasons are social-economical, then at least these people can be regarded as an at-risk subgroup, just like the elderly male with co-morbid conditions, so that they can be offered more specific protection in preparation for the next wave or future waves of outbreaks.

So with the present data that we know of, one can draw the preliminary conclusions that Asians have lower death rates, while some of the richest countries in the world (the USA and parts of the rich Europe) have much higher death rates especially in care homes and among the black population. To add to further confusion, those countries in Eastern Europe, which are much less prosperous than those in G10, all seemed to have lower numbers of cases and deaths. These countries made much earlier efforts in closing down their borders and starting social isolation, but their level of hospital services is generally regarded as less advanced. Can all these be explained by the fact that these rich countries took the appropriate healthcare actions later than others, lockdown later, tests later, isolation later? I have a suspicion that this would be too simplistic an explanation. It is almost tempting to speculate that it may be a rich country's disease. The richer the countries are, the higher the number of deaths. It defies belief, and it is counterintuitive. Can it be due to income inequality affecting the black people who actually work in low paid jobs with poor environment conditions such as those found in grey economies, where there may be no minimal wages, no proper break for rest, living in poor and overcrowded lodgings in cramped conditions and substandard hygiene? And for those in care homes, which also have high excess deaths with Covid-19, did the staff caring for these high-risk elderly people have regular training in infection control and were they properly supervised? These are very sensitive but nonetheless important issues that Covid-19 has thrown up for debate. One debate may even address the more sensitive and moral question: can it be speculated that the rich are getting richer at the expense of the poor and the elderly? To what extent are poverty and social neglect the contributing factors in the high number of deaths in the West? The answer seems to be intuitive. Clearly early figures can only serve to alert trends, and they may not lead to conclusions. Verifications are needed. These are difficult questions, but the answer for these must be sought as it will help us to cope better when the next outbreak comes. Morally, it should be in our beings that those who are vulnerable in our societies need our help most in times of crisis.

CHAPTER 14

What now?

We were all hoping that with the warmer weather in the Northern Hemisphere and with most of the heavily affected countries already past the peak of the pandemic, then perhaps the outbreak would be behind us after the summer. But this is precisely the time to ask ourselves: what next, what lessons have we learned and what do we need to unlearn, in order for us to move on, to be better prepared for the next wave of infection?

Covid-19 is a pivotal and watershed moment for us. We are at the crossroads, in trying to figure out which direction(s) we wish to travel for the next phase of human developments, and for our future generations. We have choices and decisions to make, plenty of them. To pretend otherwise would be a folly. We must press the reset button, based on what we have gone through, and reboot our thinking to build a better world for us to live in. We can choose to improve life together, which means we must trust each other by crossing national boundaries. Or, we can protect ourselves inwardly by reverting to tribal and selfish thinking while suspicious of others, thus reducing trust with each other. Globalization was already on the retreat and Covid-19 may have given this deceleration process further momentum. Countries which preached the success of globalization are now looking inwards and starting to look at self-sufficiency. East is East and West is West, and never the twain shall meet. Asians will perhaps stop eating McDonald's burgers or stop buying Prada handbags. The ordinary American citizens may not be able to buy cheap Chinese-made toys, electronics, clothes or mobile phones. The American farming belt, instead of producing corn and soya bean to be exported to China, may be converted to making masks and ventilators to protect the US public for the next wave. The road ahead would therefore be bumpy, and fragmented even. Such narrowminded, nationalistic thinking would not do anyone any good, except for the flag waving, foreigner-rejecting few in a frenzy of nationalistic fervour. The world order established after WW2 certainly was not built like that. It was built on a spirit of co-operation, a sort of never again motto after the carnage in Europe, China and Japan. The USA came to the forefront to lead the world. After WW2, fifty countries signed up to form the United Nations in San Francisco, and now the UN boasts member states comprising 193 sovereign countries. It has its faults, but it does play a role in reducing the risk of war. Covid-19 has shown us, in clear and certain terms, that we need to sit down and think seriously and rationally on a major re-evaluation of what matters to us. If there is one thing that Covid-19 taught us, then it is that we must act together and not let this virus tear us apart. We desperately need leadership, both at home and on the international stage, a leadership which understands that in the new post-Covid-19 world we have to have a common pathway. Things are indeed grim right now, but if we can ditch tribalism for the common good, then a rainbow will await us at the end of the storm. If we allow the virus to make us regress back to a disunited world, then the virus will have won, even before it hits out in the next wave. We have beaten smallpox, hepatitis and HIV, so our aim now must be to contain further waves of Covid-19 and our direction of travel does require visionary leadership from all sides.

There are three big areas which nearly all countries have to face and tackle. The more serious that countries are in addressing these, the better the chance of success and the better for the common good. The post-Covid-19 world can act as our great leveller, the great divergence becomes the great convergence in recognizing the need to be united in fighting any virus attacks in the future. Covid-19 showed us in just a few months that countries have different infections and death rates. Yet our health is equally important to us all. There needs to be a convergence of policies to fight the virus in whatever health systems we find ourselves in, by balancing national with international needs.

The global economy

It is hard to see how things will play out. The pessimists point out that the world economy will face a depression which may be much deeper than the last Great Depression in 1929. The Bank of England pointed out in May 2020 at the height of the crisis in the UK that the country's GDP for 2020 may fall as much as 14%, the biggest on record in its 300-year history. The optimists guess that while 2020 will undoubtedly be a year of negative growth, 2021 may be a year when global growth can resume. No one can be sure; either camp can be right. The only exception may be China where there may be positive growth in the second half of 2020 which may even out the recession it had in the first half of the year. China went into lockdown quicker and came out of it much quicker too in the second quarter, though the overall net growth will still be weak.

While economists use their expert knowledge and know-how in working out their projections from the economic models, we know that for each country, there was at least a period of six to eight weeks of near complete shutdown when shops were closed, people stayed at home, and the salaried people were furloughed. Economic growth depends on activity and on that basis, the outlook post-Covid-19 would be grim. All governments, whatever their ideology, including the most capitalistic of them all, the USA, have been acting big and spending big by huge amount of quantitative easing (printing money) at near zero interest rate. Such magnitude of quantitative easing does mean that all central governments will be in a heavy debt burden which will take years to pay back, but there simply is no alternative. Rebuilding the economy following Covid-19 takes time and courage to spend whatever it takes. This is the only way to help the public to survive, by putting health and lives before national budget deficit. Keeping people afloat first and then the economy hopefully can be revived by the people later. Because this is truly a once-in-a-lifetime pandemic, so for any solution to work its way through, it has to be a solution which most countries can follow and the economic impact can be shared and evened out. This same global approach should also be adopted for the coordination of research on specific antiviral drug treatment or vaccine for Covid-19. So far, it certainly appears that most governments are unanimous in this, spending whatever it takes to stop the spread. Vaccination nationalism should be avoided.

Once the viral spread has receded, then the next urgent key challenge is how to unlock and restart the economic activities. Opening up too early may risk a second wave, opening too late will cause further damage to the economy. The public may get angry either way. This is not an open and shut case and the economic recovery would not be a V-shape kind of rebound. Factories may restart but would the products be sold in the same marketplace and welcomed by the same customer as it was before Covid-19? Airlines will operate again but would there be enough passengers? Hotels will reopen but will there be enough tourists? Governments may wish to rethink their strategy and make health policy decisions so that the essential supplies will not be caught short again. Private companies will have to make totally different commercial decisions to generate growth. While we can safely assume some pharmaceuticals will make a breakthrough in antiviral treatment or vaccine, how would a reasonable price be set so that the whole world can benefit from it and not just only the rich countries? In short, while we can guess who may be the winners, how can we ensure the losers do not get left behind? These are not easy questions to answer but at least one can make a very basic assumption, which is that global recovery is only possible if there is international co-operation, goodwill and coordination. The supply chain problem may have caused difficulties in recent times, but it does not mean we need to break the whole chain. We just need to be smarter at it and not really ditching it. For the world economy to recover, the first thing to do is to guard against the overreaction to and the backlash against the perceived problems of globalization. Just-in-time has not turned overnight into a bad motto, as it does improve efficiency and avoid wastage. This motto needs to be coupled with the just-in-case motto to improve resilience. A balanced approach to both mottos internationally can bring us the much-needed economic benefits and prevent us from being caught again in the mayhem witnessed in the last nine months since the beginning of 2020, as well as help us cope better when the next wave of viral attack comes.

Politics and economy go hand in hand. The better the global politics, the better the economy, and vice versa. Regrettably, right now, the two biggest economies in the world are at loggerheads with each other. Their political ideology is different and so is their system of governance. Such is the polarisation and the schism that was opened up in the last few years that there were even, most worryingly of all, recent talks about the Thucydides Trap. Thucydides was a historian in Ancient Greece who put forward the political theory that when one great power is rising, it will inevitably threaten to displace the established power, which consistently will result in war. In this case, it means China and the USA. War between China and the USA is simply unthinkable, as the two powers are so intertwined and are co-dependent on each other. Defeat for one will cause untold damage to the other too, a pyrrhic victory indeed. These two big countries have already been engaged in a major dispute on tariffs for a good part of two years. The rest of the world, from Asia to Australasia to Europe, from Africa to South America and Canada, could only act as anxious observers rather than mediators. After intense negotiations and public relations campaign from both sides, an initial Phase I agreement was reached in January 2020. But no sooner was the ink barely dry, on came to the world stage Covid-19, which changed everything.

Because Covid-19 started in Wuhan and because there was some initial confusion in China about how best to handle this crisis, coming so close to the all-important annual Spring Festival in the country, there was this tendency in the right wing sector of the USA press to lay the blame on China, even suggesting some sort of human conspiracy from the laboratory. Some countries and press jumped onto this bandwagon, which in turn compelled China to defend itself. Seeing itself as grossly misunderstood and unfairly treated with groundless criticisms, China, as the first victim of the outbreak, shared with the rest of the world openly the moment it cracked the

RNA sequence of Cov9d-19, even before it was designated as Covid-19 by the WHO. China sees this as an honest and goodwill gesture. It is non-proprietary, so that the rest of the world can work for a diagnostic test, a treatment and a vaccine. China felt hard done to. This goodwill was never properly appreciated in the public press, though it was appreciated in the international scientific community.

In my view, perhaps this rising tension and war of words can galvanize the cool heads to return to the front of the debate. The lesson to learn here is Covid-19 attacks everyone, that is the very nature of a viral attack. At this time of international crisis, we must unlearn nationalism as it almost certainly will impede our efforts to rekindle the global economy and our global efforts in coming up with treatments and vaccines. In short, international political co-operation needs to be the working model. Nationalism, even if exists in only some quarters, should be parked aside and not allowed to get in the way.

Once international co-operation is agreed and assured, then the next step is for the international financial sector, mainly the banks, to come to the rescue with governments making significant loan guarantees. Unlike the last crisis in 2008, which was created by the financial sector, this time round, the financial sector can really come to the rescue of the public and business sector by providing liquidity. The central banks, which are the banks of last resort, all over the world, have already lowered the base lending rate to an unprecedented level, so the commercial banks can afford to borrow to lend to the various businesses to keep them afloat, at least to give them a fighting chance to recover as the viral attack recedes. The worst outcome is when the viral attack has receded, there is no variable business left, especially small-to-medium businesses! The people who may want to go out for a birthday dinner or married couples wanting to go abroad for a honeymoon may find that there are limited restaurants to go to or flights to book. These services are there to serve ordinary people. If these services go under, it would mean the remaining services will be servicing only the rich, but even the rich, if a vicious cycle of spiralling downwards is allowed to happen, may not be so rich after all. The time has also now come for the banks not to think about the interests of the shareholders but more the customers, who either are depositors or borrowers. If shareholders' dividends are cut, then at least there is a chance the dividends will come at a later time when the economy does recover. Everyone can and should bear some pain to help the others. In the UK, some big companies such as HSBC and British Telecom have already announced they will not pay out dividends, on the government's advice. One would expect that there will be an outcry on this from the investors, especially the big institutional investors such as pension funds, but so far, there have not been any major criticisms coming out from any quarters.

Business confidence is one of the key requirements needed for economic growth. If the business sector is confident that liquidity is forthcoming, then they will worry less about insolvency but concentrate more on maintaining or even expanding their business, and modify their business to fit in with the new normal. This is just like the medical scenario in a dehydrated patient from a hard day of exhaustion in the hottest of weather; he will need a careful intravenous drip, and as long as he is on an intravenous drip for rehydration, then he can be reasonably confident of survival and recovery. Once the IV drip is off, he can be discharged and at some stage he would be a fully productive member of society. Illness is often treatable if the right medicine is administered, so currently, public health measures and financial support are the right medicine to help us to get onto the road to economic recovery while we all wait for new and better medicine to come.

In short, the global recovery will need coordinated monetary policy of the governments to ensure active assistance from the banking sector to the business sector, so that the business sector and the public can make plans to realign the business and customer behaviour with the new normal to revive the economy.

The New Normal

The new normal is here to stay, and we have to be prepared
not only to accept it, but to support and be part of it too.
The new normal should be a new way of life to which the
public and the business community all need to adapt. The
reason for this is simple. It has in its origin as to how our
social behaviour can be modified in such a way to reduce
the chance of cross-infection. In other words, personal
hygiene and public hygiene standards will be raised to a
new standard. The advantage of this is not only will it help
us to deal with the next wave of Covid-19, or 21 or 23, as the
case may be, it will also protect us from other infections,
such as TB or any other infections transmissible by droplets.
Awareness of the importance of hygiene and thus changing
our behaviour accordingly is arguably one of the best
things that we have learned while coming out of Covid-19.
At the height of the outbreak in China, I often talked to my
colleagues about this. We all agreed, without exception,
that it would be so wasteful if we do not learn from this
experience. Nearly all countries were caught short and this
lesson will give the world, the governments and the people
a real chance of living a different, healthier and recalibrated
life. New economic growth is welcome, but it would be
meaningless if the growth is only measured by the same
headline-grabbing stories such as the speed of the recovery,

government deficits, unemployment rate or GDP. Growth has to be seen in a way that other factors can be considered too and that future shocks of another outbreak can be cushioned. Would it be too far-fetched to suggest a GHI (global health index) or GHP (global happiness product), in addition to GDP?

When China was going through the peak of the crisis, there were pictures and articles in the press of how the pollution index was much better and thus the quality of air was better. A perverse argument then came forward that a crisis was needed to improve the environment. Now this is a view too far-fetched and even irresponsible. The crisis occurred out of the blue, no one was expecting it and the reason for the cleaner and better air was explainable by the complete lockdown of the cities and cessation of economic activities such as factory productions. The virus was there to infect humans, not with the intention of making air cleaner. This, however, may give us a chance to think outside the box. We know the new normal compels us to work differently and minimal physical distance from each other needs to be maintained, even in situations where there are crowds such as sporting events or musical concerts. We can now learn from what the supermarkets are doing, we can now see how quiet and peaceful the GP practices are, and will come to the conclusion that the way these services are refigured has not caused us significant inconvenience, and in fact, none. We still get what we need, though it may take a bit longer. But we trade this with a better and safer environment for us to live and work in.

In the near future, we need to consider those working in offices, especially the civil services. Can the working hours be rearranged in such a way that the work attendance is based on teams and that not everyone is rushing to work between 8 a.m. and 9 a.m.? This could make time for those who need to take their children to school and later pick them up. This arrangement can reduce the congestion in peak times and even reduce air pollution from traffic congestion. In the UK, the government used car activity as a daily index of the effects of lockdown. And the data clearly showed that the carbon footprint is much less. In London, there is now already talk of car-free zones which may replace the congestion charge, a charge which the rich with a Porsche undoubtedly have no problem paying, however punitive the charge may be. Furthermore, would the government take a lead in this new normal by piloting that the civil service working hours be split into day and evening time, so that those with work and children at school would probably not need to rush all the time? Before Covid-19, our life was split and structured into daytime, which for most people is either work or school, and evening time, which for most is rest or homework. As such, activities are all congested in the daytime, thus increasing the risk of cross-infection as well as increasing the carbon footprint in the day. Is there a need for a government-led task force to look at the ways in which the day can be split into several flexible parts to serve the need of the workers, balancing it with the need to protect society from infection? We can take a lesson here from the people who work in the emergency services or the essential services. They are used to working on shifts. Let us, for argument's sake, ask them for a view if they are all willing to go back to a non-shift pattern of work. My sneaky suspicion is that their answer may surprise us all, as they would probably prefer to stay working shifts. This will give us further scope in exploring how we can make real adjustments out of this new normal.

The Earth works in the same way for all of us. We all have the same 24 hours every day. We should ask ourselves how we define a normal day. What is the normal working time when half of the world's population may be sleeping and resting while the other half of the world's population may be working? The Earth does not modify its rotation to suit us, but we adjust our life to suit the rotation. We do know there are some things which can only be done in daylight, such as farming, agriculture and gardening. But, look at the stockbrokers in the trading floors or financial analysts in the stock markets – they are so used to watching other markets in a different time zone. Those who work in London financial markets are just as stressed in the evening as in the day as the other markets may still be trading. It used to be said that the lives of these traders are easily burnt out because they have to keep an eye on what the global markets are doing on a 24-hour basis, not a second and the smallest piece of information can be missed, or they would either lose the chance of making more money or actually risk losing money. On the other hand, look at the ambulance crew, fire crew or the police, their stress is not whether they are on duty or not but the stress starts when someone is suddenly ill, when a fire breaks out or a crime committed. Illness, fire and crime do not happen round the clock, most of them happen by accident and sporadically. That is, the timing of fire and crime may be unpredictable, but their work and rest time are predictable. So is it entirely possible that we reassess our conventional working hours and re-evaluate our lives to adjust to the post Covid-19 world? Can we think about spreading out our working hours a bit more, say from 8 a.m. to 9 p.m. (in two shifts) over a 24-hour period? Where is the rule book that said clerical office hours have to be 9 a.m. to 5 p.m.? The spreading out can help us not only to continue to practise social distancing to prevent infection but also bring about less congestion which would help to achieve a more eco-friendly environment. For instance, a recent study from Peking University has shown that in Beijing, the average usage of the subways is now much lower at the weekends, compared with weekdays. There was a sharp difference in 2020 compared with 2019. This may suggest the emergence of a new normal trend that people may prefer going to work during the week to going out for leisure during the weekend. In fact, for most people, work is a form of socializing too because that is when we are meeting our colleagues, and some may become our friends. So this may prompt the municipal administration to pilot a rearrangement of a normal working day and working week for office workers. The same problem of congestion in the subway can be seen in Tokyo, London and Hong Kong. In fact, the rush hour human congestion in the subways of these cities has to be seen to be believed. One look at the congestion will put anyone off from getting onto the trains in these days of collective public vigilance to prevent viral infection. Rearrangement of work to offload the peak time congestion will help to reduce risk of cross-infection further.

Covid-19 is a transformative event for the world. The magnitude and the speed of its attack shocked us all, many people died and the fear is that the new waves will come. We just don't know where or when. We, over the past few months, have made adjustments in the way we live and do things differently and now gradually we see the emergence of this new normal. We now have a choice. We can either wait till Covid-19 fully recedes and choose to go back to our old way, and forget everything that had happened and see Covid-19 as nothing but a bad dream from which we have just woken up. That would be a very easy and tempting thing to do, but over years, complacency will set in again as old habits die hard while the next wave and the wave after will keep setting us back. The alternative is to take stock and have a serious debate on what we have learned from the painful experiences we have been put through. We must face up to the hard lesson this virus has taught us in this once-in-a-lifetime experience, and we must try not to be caught again when the next wave comes! The decision we make in the next year or so would have profound impact on our children, and our children's children.

I believe in the triumph of the human spirit. The new normal is our way of protecting our future generations. It will take years to get the new normal to be part of our behaviour culture. It will require courage and perseverance, not only on an individual level, but at a community level, a national level, and in a perfect world, at international level. Could this be the time the great divergence becomes the great convergence when all of us can have the same approach in living our daily lives, when the words such as East and West will only have a geographical connotation but not a political one?

The next wave

It is generally agreed by all scientists and epidemiologists that the next wave of attack will come, that is part of the biology and evolution of a viral attack. The only thing we do not know is when and where. The thing we could know, or at least make a real attempt to, is what to do when the next wave does come. One can use a real life example to illustrate the point. Since 1945, we all knew what the destructive power of an atomic bomb is. It was a real demonstration of the power of a weapon of mass destruction (WMD). We also know, from the calculations by the nuclear physicists, how modern day nuclear arsenals can be so much more destructive than those old atomic bombs. That is what we know. What we don't know is how and when and where it will be used. Because it will cause massive destruction, it serves as a natural deterrent to the humans deploying the same WMD again. It makes those countries which possess nuclear weapons very cautious, as they all know that their adversaries can retaliate by using the same weapons. This is called mutual assured destruction (MAD) and it is the single most powerful reason that since 1945, we have not seen its use, and continue to pray that we will never see it used. Because of the sheer power of the theory of MAD, it has led the world to have a nuclear non-proliferation treaty, and arms control talks. Even without further expansion in the existing arsenal, the current nuclear weapons can guarantee that we can destroy planet Earth many, many times over, at the press of a few buttons. So those with the control buttons have built in layers of safety valves, and cool heads always prevail when the temperature runs high. We have seen wars since 1945, we have seen many lives lost from wars too since 1945, but at least we have never seen the nuclear button being pressed again. Some say that the atomic bomb in Hiroshima is the single reason why there is no third world war. Long may this be continued.

This proved that the international community can work together to prevent the apocalyptic nuclear button from being pressed, despite the ideological differences and hostilities between nations and despite the hot headed rhetoric, the tendency to issue threats and treat each other as adversaries. Covid-19 may be erroneously portrayed by some as a weapon, but the fact is, it is a virus and the outbreak was an act of nature. What we do need to be mindful of is that it is certain to come back again and again to cause us untold sufferings and inconvenience. Every time this happens, it would be a human crisis and not merely a national crisis. So the international communities have a duty to work and fight together against the invisible but guaranteed threat from this virus to prevent the carnage we have witnessed in 2020. Covid-19 had killed around 672,000 worldwide by July 2020. Since the world has already signed up for the control of man-made biological or chemical warfare, there is all the more reason to do the same for naturally occurring viral infection. We were successful in eradicating smallpox, in controlling HIV and hepatitis, so let us turn our attention to Covid-19. Discussions in previous chapters centred on our efforts on economic measures and our way of coping with the new normal; the third essential ingredient is how to prevent, or ameliorate, the next wave of attack when it comes.

On balance, I am optimistic on this. I come to this view as I recalled how quickly China shared the RNA sequencing in early January with the rest of the world. In any fight against any virus, the first battle has always been to know the genomics of the virus. This sharing of information was a move which transcended national boundaries or any debate on intellectual property. I have always felt knowledge is only true knowledge when it is shared and not possessed. If we cast our mind back to the early 1980s when the HIV story first broke, the medical community was struggling with why, until it was found out and proved almost 10 years later that it was caused by a virus.

The first battle was won, at great cost, in knowing the RNA sequence of Covid-19 and getting the outbreak under control through unredeemed lockdown measures. The war, however, has not been won, far from it.

The second battle to be won is on information sharing. To win the war on Covid-19, it requires, certainly within the scientific and academic circles, great determination to work together, to speed up the learning process, pooling information all over the world. Within five months of the attack by Covid-19, there were already clinical trials, not only national clinical trials but also international trials, some coordinated by the WHO, using a single drug or a combination of drugs, plasma products from recovered patients, or even traditional Chinese medicine. Nothing was ruled out. It matters not in my view if results of some of these trials initially proved disappointing. No one could hit the bull's eye in the first go. The progress of medicine is not like a straight flight of an arrow in its predictable trajectory, but always full of ups and downs, twists and turns. The urgency of scientific and clinical validations of these results, the ethical consideration of the merits of the trials, and the rapid dissemination of the results to share with the world have to have the collective support of governments, the regulatory bodies and the prestigious international journals, all ready to fast track the work by cutting out bureaucracy. The example I wish to quote is the role of the journal *Lancet*. *Lancet* is a world famous journal of outstanding international fame and respect. This journal is first off the block to give those who worked in this crisis a platform. It is such a highly respected platform that everyone takes notice when *Lancet* makes a stand. *Lancet* for many years has enjoyed its long distinguished tradition of being scientifically cautious and impartial before publishing, but given the urgency and the enormous global impact this crisis may have on the whole world, *Lancet* took a stand on Covid-19 and decided to fast track peer reviewed clinical information for publication. When *Lancet* makes a stand, the whole world takes notice. If there is a Pulitzer prize in medical journals as there is in the newspaper industry, then I think *Lancet* would have won hands down in 2020, and deservedly so too. By providing such a powerful platform, it gives people working in this field the extra motivation to fight the disease, since they know that they can share the fruits of their labour on a platform of international repute, even if their good work may not bring about the desired result. There are of course some people, whom I would call the traditionalists, who take a slightly negative view of the stand of *Lancet*. The noises from these quarters are totally missing the point. This is a global crisis and the whole world needs to take note. The stance that *Lancet* takes to give Covid-19 its prominence is to give this global public health crisis the highest international priority it has fully merited. It may not win a Nobel Prize, but it will be a huge recognition for the humanitarian efforts in this. Governments as a result were ready to turn on the green light and fast track the scientific and clinical endeavours, mainly because of the messages coming out from *Lancet*, which has been tireless in its effort to work with global communities to stress the seriousness of Covid-19.

Now, even though the virus can attack humans, it can no longer attack us in secret. Our second battle was won on information sharing. That this key second battle was won is due to the combinations of various factors. The first factor is the openness and the extensive coverage on Covid-19 by the respectable press in the world. Unlike *Lancet*, which is a professional peer reviewed journal, the press is for the public even though, like *Lancet*, the public can only get access to this respectable press by subscription. However, due to the global and serious nature of the outbreak, one does not need to be a subscriber to read all these newspapers. Most international press is now providing readers with free, electronic-based Covid-19 information. The second factor is the way the clinicians and scientists chose to seize the initiatives in sharing what they know and what they want to know by submitting their opinions and data to peer reviewed journals, on a fast track net-based platform, in addition to journals like *Lancet*. This also has an additional effect of further motivating and uniting the professionals working on Covid-19 from various countries to share information. The third factor is the use of technology in tracking the virus and location of the clusters of outbreak in a local community, such as what is seen in China, to help us to know, as the public, where the virus is and thus we can keep a distance from it.

The third battle is how to stop the next wave in its tracks before it hits us. We have to nip it in the bud. Since the virus knows no boundary, we humans should not have boundaries too in fighting it. At this stage, the world generally knows what to do. Measures such as social distancing and self-isolation have proven their effectiveness. Furthermore, we now have enough information, which came out within a few months of the start of Covid-19, that some people are far more vulnerable to this virus with a higher death rate. These are the elderly, those living in care homes, and those with a poorer social economic background, especially black people in the advanced economies of the West. Governments can then make the appropriate risk-targeted policies to protect these groups.

The final battle to win the war is of course by stopping the virus from infecting humans or preventing it from re-emerging altogether. For this to be achieved, there are specific areas we must work on. These areas are vital to our success.

We need to resolve the issue of tests. As mentioned previously, there are needs for two types of tests. The present confusion must be cleared up and the difficulties must be overcome. The first hurdle is that those who claim to provide the tests must have the scientific integrity to make sure the tests are accurate, precise, valid and reproducible. The integrity of these providers, some of whom may be upstart entrepreneurs but most of them are already part of a large multinational pharmaceutical, should be at the top of the agenda at a time when the whole world is looking at them for solutions. At this time of crisis, it is never more important that ethics and integrity should be uppermost in their consideration, along with the technological ability. This is especially so since nearly all governments have shown a real act of good faith in fast tracking approvals, and so these suppliers of such tests must not take advantage of this by behaving irresponsibly. Their primary motivation should not be the sale figures but efficacy and serving the public without the obsession to race to the top of the fame and profit league. If they do, they betray the trust the public has placed on them just when the public is at its most vulnerable. As an example of ethics and standards, I would like to highlight what the government in China did. In April 2020, the whole world was chasing the suppliers of the test. The UK government was also desperate in looking for a test, as there was already widespread criticism against the UK government in the slowness of its uptake of the test. There was, however, another side to the caution and the deliberation by the UK government. Even though it was true that the diagnostic abilities of the UK as a country have fallen behind other countries, precautions were exercised by the professionals in upholding the principle that one must not rush to do the test for the sake of it unless one is reasonably sure of the validity of the test. Spain, another country heavily hit by Covid-19, announced also in April 2020 that it was sending some test kits for Covid-19 back to the suppliers in China. This gave the press an opportunity to write and condemn the practice of the suppliers in China for a substandard product, in a classic example of one swallow does make a spring. This negative press was a deserved criticism. This was a real alert at the time, as it actually injected a degree of realistic caution to the panic buyers. It later turned out that the specific supplier was not on the approval list of tests in China for export; the supplier was only waiting to be approved. Following that development, the Chinese government made a worldwide announcement. It stated that anyone exporting any tests or materials for Covid-19-related products must first undertake to seek a proper approval from the country that the products are exported to. I thought that was a very smart move, a very fair move too. Since all countries have border control and that people from a different country must have an entry visa before being allowed in, why should health products such as tests for a virus not have a similar entry visa too? The risk is now shared by both sides, the provider and the buyer. Suppose

I find myself to have some fever and cough, I may want to rush to buy the first kit, perhaps even the most expensive kit, that is available in the drug store. I may base my choice on seeing the advertisements, often displayed in Google or Amazon, informing me that a new, quick diagnostic test is now available at the pinprick of a finger or a cotton swab in my throat, without needing any training, and that this test will have the ability to tell me within an hour the reason for my fever. All the providers need to do is put a disclaimer in mini print in the kit handout to absolve them of their sloppiness. But whether I can really be reassured by the result of this point-of-care testing to guide my next actions is of course open to doubt. Just because it is new, easy to use, and can satisfy my anxious need to know, does not necessarily mean it is valid and accurate.

This is precisely the reason why caution should be exercised, even more so in times of crisis. A cool head is needed in a hot-headed environment. Advertisements are no more or no less than just advertisements. It is in their nature to highlight the good without mentioning the not-so-good. The message therefore can be best summed up for the test providers as follows: Now the government has fast tracked and opened up all the channels, so bureaucracy hurdles can no longer be used as an excuse. The public is vulnerable, so you, as manufacturers of these tests or materials, must fulfil your obligations in upholding the highest professional and ethical standards. This principle should apply equally to both the big world-famous diagnostic giants and the upstarts; reputation may count but validity counts even more. In the final analysis, the governments can resort to the power bestowed on them by their people in fining or banning these providers, in much the same way a drunk driver has his licence taken away.

The next thing to move on from the test is the treatment of those who have the infection. Here again, caution and openness are the key. There are early reports that some existing drugs on the market for conditions other than viral infection are effective and while the jury is out on its efficacy, the world then rapidly runs out of supplies of these drugs. My own bet on this is that success in treating this virus is more likely on the work currently undertaken on specific antiviral drugs, based on the experience of HIV treatment and hepatitis B treatment. In other words, just like antibiotics and other viral treatments, they must be targeted specifically against the living organisms. There are now many well-designed clinical trials conducted all over the world, mainly in advanced economies. Some of these are national trials, particularly those conducted in the USA. Most are multinational trials, under the auspices of either big international pharmaceutical companies or the WHO. Every bit of information coming out of this will be scrutinized; even negative information is better than no

information. It is a matter of huge regret that at the times
of SARS and MERS, many early promises were made to
find an effective antiviral treatment, but as SARS and
MERS somehow mysteriously disappeared, so went the
effort to find the effective treatment. In retrospect, had
those earlier promises been honoured, there was every
chance a treatment would have been found then. Given that
Covid-19, SARS and MERS are all part of the same family
of coronaviruses, the same treatment used previously
might well be effective for Covid-19 and the world would
not be so badly caught, or have paid such a high human or
economical price. In 2003 and again in 2012, an opportunity
for finding a specific antiviral treatment was hugely missed
and the lesson must be learned. It was also a case where
the big pharmaceuticals decided, for commercial reasons,
that since the outbreak had subsided, there were no clinical
demands for such a drug and no profits could be made, so
no need to go down that manufacturing road. It would be
better to concentrate on drugs for cancer and heart diseases.
Capitalism and the free market have always been reputed
to be the best at allocation of resources. This was like a slap
in the face for those who show blind faith in capitalism
and the role of the market. Blind faith is just as bad as no
faith, just like a wrong test is as bad as no test. Now the
pandemic has shown us that by September 2020 the total
number of affected cases has reached beyond 30 million,

with the richest country in the world having the largest number of cases. The potential demand will be globally unprecedented. The market and profitability for the big pharmaceutical companies will be huge, since every expert in the world is now predicting there will be a second wave or even a third wave. This market is clearly enticing for the big pharmaceutical players. I am not for any minute here condemning this aspect of capitalism and the free market. I fully accept and understand that the big pharmaceutical companies are there to help cure diseases and should be rewarded, given the massive investments they all have made in developing new drugs. I am simply pointing out the principle of 'do good work first, then fame and fortune will come, not the other way round'. The heart should be in the right place to direct the brain. On this point, I am overall optimistic that effective treatment will come as long as we continue to make the effort and not repeat the same mistake as in SARS and MERS. At the time of writing this book, the front runner for the specific antiviral treatment of Covid-19 is remdesivir. It has been approved by the UK regulator for its clinical use. Initial evidence showed that it can shorten the time to recovery though no overall survival benefit can be demonstrated as yet. More clinical information will have to be collected before any rational conclusion can be drawn. The standard recommendation of a five-day course will cost around GBP 2,000.

The final key part in our third battle against Covid-19 when we aim to win the war is the development of vaccines. Edward Jenner is still considered as the founder of vaccinology when, in 1796, after he inoculated a 13-year-old boy with the vaccinia virus, commonly known as cowpox, he demonstrated immunity to smallpox in this young boy. Two years later, in 1798, the first smallpox vaccine was developed, with the result that the war against smallpox was won by massive vaccination, and smallpox was declared to be eradicated globally in 1979 by the WHO, just under 200 years later – in the year that I got my licence to practise as a medical doctor. It left such a deep impression on me as at that time, freshly qualified as a young and inexperienced doctor, I had never heard of an infectious disease being eradicated. Before that, smallpox carried a mortality of 30% and even higher in babies. The story of smallpox must be remembered, as it can always be an inspiration for those of us who deal with diseases.

Of course, medical science has advanced beyond all imagination and expectations in the intervening years. Genetics was not regarded as a proper science until the 19th century when the Austrian Gregor Mendel made a science of it by studying inheritance through observing pea plants. Then in the 20th century, in 1953, Watson and Crick discovered the double helix, thus laying the foundation for our understanding of genes and genomics.

All these steps help us to move forward, step by step, successes alternating with failures, in our effort to truly prevent or even eradicate a disease by vaccination, from smallpox to measles to hepatitis. Vaccination and immunization are very complex processes, requiring scientific input from all areas, not least those at the forefront of science, the patients, the volunteers and the doctors. This group of people would allow us to directly benefit from the sweet fruits of success of science. I may feel, once again, if a vaccine is developed for Covid-19, the joy I had years ago at hearing of the eradication of smallpox. The research efforts and the resources invested internationally in developing this vaccine are, in my lifetime, unparalleled. Because Covid-19 is such an unforgiving pandemic, fighting it has moved to the top of the international agenda. All countries, without exception, have pledged support and co-operation. At the time of writing this manuscript, there are 11 candidate vaccines, according to the WHO, which have reached the stage of clinical testing. The WHO says that only Oxford University's vaccine has reached what is known as Phase 3, the final and largest-scale trial, followed by one which is being developed and tested in China, one in the USA and one in Germany.

The importance of an effective vaccine cannot be overstated but still a note of caution is needed here. We all have high hopes that the first vaccine, by all accounts, may be available for selected high risk patients or front line healthcare workers in late 2020 or early 2021, but it must also be pointed out that the availability of a few vaccines does not guarantee their success and clinical effectiveness. It will take time, thorough and ongoing clinical studies, possibly even two to three years, to really assess the level and the sustainability of the antibody response in those who receive the vaccine. Only then will we know how to use the vaccine properly to offer us the maximal protection against Covid-19. Expectations must be managed in this respect.

With all our high hopes and noble aspirations for better health and a changed society, a note of caution and reality check must be made. In May 2020, the European Union showed commendable leadership hosting an international meeting to raise funds to speed up the efforts in fighting this virus, and to ensure that populations, both rich and poor, have equitable access. In May 2020 the funds raised were about USD 8 billion, pledged by governments, big pharmaceutical companies and private donors. The sum estimated to actually make a vaccine is about three times that much. But the funding required for a vaccine, huge as it may sound, is a modest commitment compared to the economic cost of the pandemic. So the development of vaccines is very cost effective. Regrettably, countries such as the USA, India and Russia did not take part in these initiatives. I hope they will get on board soon. In the short term, all governments will be torn between priorities to test, to treat or to invest in vaccines. All three are self-evidently important, but clearly the best long-term solution is a vaccine. Tough decisions will have to be made. What is worrying is that there is an early emergence of 'vaccine nationalism'. Countries, including the USA and UK, are providing support for researchers and companies and even production within their national borders, sometimes accompanied by requirements to provide preferential access to their own citizens. Putting aside the moral and ethical side of such an approach, this could also backfire as other countries may choose to follow suit, thus the poor countries will be left unattended and denied the access to vaccine. Not only that, how could it be that a single country can launch such a vaccine with the production capacity to supply the whole world? There must be collaboration. Some countries in the key supply and production chains, which are equally important as a legitimate stakeholder, may choose to have their own national preference as well, for their own citizens. So not only the global good will be slowed down, it also may lead to further squabbles, and the final decisive battle against an invisible virus will be a stalemate right before the finishing line. This rush to be the sole winner, a rush to claim fortune and fame, should not be allowed to happen, nor should the previously unheard-of term called vaccine nationalism. We must aim for the smallpox story version 2, 2020 and never let the notion of vaccine nationalism get beyond the stage of wishful thinking. A small piece of RNA not only can infect and kill some of us, it may even claim to win in the ultimate battle before a single vaccine is given if we humans decide to start a race against each other by fighting on the front of vaccine nationalism and not against the RNA.

Never before in my lifetime is political leadership beyond borders more important, more needed and more urgent. It is not only about the triumphs of the human spirit, but the very real nobility and high ideals of our very beings. When we look up and look forward, we must not forget those who are behind or below us. We must have the faith that the world, at whatever point in its history, always has more good people than not so good people. We can be very firm in this belief, as in our daily life, we can feel for ourselves that there are far more good people than bad people. There are bad or sad stories in the press, only because good news tends to go unreported and good deeds are not so newsworthy. Our good deeds will ensure that we, the human race, will continue to advance. To conclude, as an eternal optimist and idealist, I believe we will succeed.

'For whom the bell tolls, it tolls for thee'
Ernest Hemingway 1940

www.ingramcontent.com/pod-product-compliance
Lightning Source LLC
Chambersburg PA
CBHW070925210326
41520CB00021B/6812